Limbic Reflexology
Student Textbook
Revised Edition

Hamish Edgar

Limbic Reflexology
Student Textbook
Revised Edition

Copyright © 2018 Hamish Edgar

Acknowledgements

My journey with Limbic has dominated my life and my thoughts since 2011. It has been punctuated with periods of confusion and frustration, periods of elation and eureka moments, and little by little, the jigsaw has revealed itself.

My gratitude and thanks go to family and friends who throughout all this have encouraged and supported me, none more so than Jan, who has been my sounding board and has endured endless soliloquies in my quest to find answers.

I must thank all my clients for their invaluable contribution in developing limbic, and who have often shared with me some of those eureka moments. Without them, Limbic would not have happened. My thanks especially to Andrew for his insights, inspiration, humour and encouragement.

Finally, my gratitude to Vicky Laws and Louise Greenwood, my tutors at the start of my reflexology journey, and to the Limbic students who have shared this Limbic journey with me. Their feedback and suggestions have been invaluable in the evolution of Limbic and the Limbic Reflexology Course. I thank them all for embracing Limbic Reflexology and taking my baby out there.

Contents

Acknowledgements i

Preface to first edition vi

Preface to the revised edition vii

Introduction viii

Limbic Reflexology Training xi

How to use this book xiii

Limbic Reflexology view of the brain. xv

The Limbic Brain 1

The Gross Structure of the Brain 3

Cells of the Central Nervous System 7

Chemical Synapse 11

Receptors 15

Neurotransmitters 16

The Limbic Brain Nuclei and Reflex Areas 21

    Insula or Insular Cortex 23

    Amygdala 27

    Hippocampus. 31

    Subiculum. 34

Locus Coeruleus 35

Thalamus 39

Striatum. 43

Nucleus Accumbens 45

Orbitofrontal Cortex 47

Subgenual Anterior Cingulate 49

Pituitary 51

Hypothalamus 53

Paraventricular Nucleus (PVN) 55

Preoptic Nucleus (PO) 56

Lateral Hypothalamus Nucleus (LHA) 57

Tuberomammillary Nucleus (TMN) 58

Suprachiasmatic Nucleus (SCN) 59

Mammillary Bodies(MB) 60

Bed Nucleus of the Stria Terminalis (BNST) 62

Periaqueductal Grey (PAG) 66

Raphe Nucleus. 68

Substantia Nigra / VTA 70

Cingulate Cortex 72

Corpus Callosum 77

Midline Thalamus 78

Reuniens (RE)..78

Habenula & Pineal 80

Cerebellum..82

Stress - a challenge to homeostasis. 84

The Stress Response 86

HPA Axis...86

Eustress and Distress 92

General Adaptation Syndrome 92

Emotions and how they arise. 96

Memory & Learning 98

Types of Memory..102

Encoding 103

Storage...103

Consolidation 103

Retrieval...104

'Sins' of memory 104

Pain...110

The Physiology of Pain 112

Pain Inhibition..117

Emotion and perception of pain 124

Pain and the Limbic Brain 127

Chronic Pain 131

Central Sensitisation 133

Mindfulness and Meditation 136

Networks. 138

Saliency Network 138

Default Mode Network and Central Executive Network .138

Common Conditions 140

Sleep 140

Anxiety 142

Depression 144

Post Trauma Stress 148

Fibromyalgia 152

Myalgic Encephalomyelitis 154

Irritable Bowel Syndrome 155

Neuropathic Pain and Complex Regional Pain Syndrome
....156

Chronic Back Pain 157

Osteoarthritis 158

Rheumatoid Arthritis 158

Glossary 160

Appendix A 162

   Medication commonly prescribed for chronic pain
   conditions. 162

Check Your Understanding. 164

Limbic Reflexology Courses 168

Index 170

Preface to first edition

In 2011, I discovered a reflex area that when worked, had a significant effect on anxiety and the somatic symptoms of anxiety. At the time I had no idea of the identity of the reflex area. Two months later, when I was reading an article about the placebo effect and the Amygdala, the Amygdala became a possible contender. However, when looking at the brain, the position of the reflex area was much too high to be the Amygdala. With further study I concluded that it was the Insula reflex area. This was confirmed by correlating symptoms and effects in others where the reflex area featured.

There remained a problem though. If this was the Insula, the Amygdala should be directly below it. The Amygdala was still too high in relation to the Pituitary reflex area. It was only when I tilted the brain back by 45 degrees that everything seemed to be in the 'right' place. Others appeared where they should be, and Limbic was born.

Still it seemed forced. Why tilt? Straightening the great toe of course tilts it back from its natural position, but that too seemed an explanation forced to fit.

It was only when I was studying the development of the embryonic brain that I discovered that at around eight week's gestation, the brain bends at 45 degrees forward at the level of the midbrain. Now I had some justification for the tilt and a tilt at that level. Tilted back to its pre-eight-weeks angle gave me the orientation of the Limbic Reflexology brain.

November 2016

Preface to the revised edition

Limbic Reflexology has evolved and will continue to do so. Over the years, I have made modifications to existing Reflex Areas in the light of experience and added others when I was confident of their identity, and as new Reflex Areas made themselves known they have been incorporated into Limbic.

Because of the evolving nature of Limbic Reflexology, keeping up to date has been a problem for past students, requiring reattendance on practical training events with the logistical problems and cost that that incurs. With the advent of Limbic Reflexology Online, an evergreen course, updating need no longer be a problem.

This revised edition includes those Reflex Areas that have emerged since 2016. I have also taken the opportunity of correcting or clarifying some material. My thanks to those who have brought these to my attention. I have been hugely encouraged by the constructive feedback about the Textbook and have incorporated many of those suggestions into this edition.

November 2018

Introduction

The limbic brain is what allows us to laugh and cry, to feel pain and fear, to control fear and pain, to enjoy music and understand humour. It allows us to feel hunger and feel that hunger satisfied.

It allows us to feel warmth and cold. It gives us our sense of being separate from others. It determines our sexuality. It gives our motivation and initiates our movement and controls all our physiological processes. It monitors our environment and initiates our responses to those changes going on around us.

Above all, the limbic brain strives to maintain homeostasis and keep us safe. In short, it is our survival machine.

Of course, the limbic brain is not exclusive to humans. It pre-dates humans. We share it with all vertebrate beings. The pattern of our limbic brain is no different to that of a hedgehog or a mouse or a fly. All the vertebrate species alive today owe their existence to being in possession of biological processes that respond to their environment in such a way, that ensures their survival. The limbic brain is at the centre of the story of evolution.

Neuroscience is an extremely complex subject and much of the brain physiology is yet poorly understood. It is important to state at the outset that it is not my intention to explain neuroscience. Rather it is about how neuroscience can inform our practice as Limbic Reflexologists.

As Reflexologists we do not need to know all about biochemistry or the intricate process of signal transduction. All this book attempts to do is to get some understanding of the principles involved in neural networks, the relevant processes, and a familiarity with the nuclei for which we can identify a corresponding reflex area.

Throughout, I have retained the conventional names of nuclei and processes. You will be unfamiliar with most of them, but once familiar, it will make scientific articles more accessible to you. This is important as part of the course involves researching a condition using scientific article and in formulating an appropriate treatment plan for a client presenting with that condition.

To be effective, the more understanding we have of neural processes the more informed and effective our treatments will be. Without that understanding, when the feet talk to us, we won't understand one word of it.

We may not yet be able to offer an acceptable explanation about 'how' reflexology works, but we can demonstrate that our practice is informed, and evidence based in terms of an understanding of the anatomy and physiology that we aim to influence.

Learning Limbic Reflexology is demanding but this is matched by the rewards of your efforts. Many who have completed the course tell me that Limbic has taken their practice to a new level. I am confident that it will do the same for you.

Hamish Edgar

November 2016

x

Limbic Reflexology Training

Limbic Reflexology was primarily intended as continued professional development for Reflexologists, but it can be incorporated into a range of other modalities.

The original training began in April 2013 in Sheffield. Since then it has evolved in content structure and delivery, with the addition of Limbic Reflexology Online in 2018.

This Textbook aims to provide familiarisation with the nuclei and processes that we aim to influence in Limbic Reflexology and the location of the reflex areas corresponding to those nuclei. It explores the anatomy and physiology of the human brain and Its central role in maintaining homeostatic norms. We explore the neurology underpinning learning and memory, mood, anxiety and fear, pain and chronic pain. Finally, we look at the limbic influence in some common conditions and problems that we encounter in our work.

In both the live and online courses, you learn the precise location of the reflex areas and the practical application of the techniques used in Limbic Reflexology.

You acquire the skills in formulating an optimum treatment plan for a given condition using credible research articles. These articles provide insights into the altered brain processes thought to be involved in those conditions, and this knowledge underpins the rationale for a treatment plan.

There are links to appropriate scientific articles in the Student Area on the limbic website, which will supplement course material.

On both courses, submission of case studies is required. In the case studies, you combine our knowledge base and practical skills. When you work the reflex areas, you will be able to make an informed interpretation of the probable dysfunctional processes underlying the client's problem and using outcome measures, introduced in the courses, you will be able to monitor changes in these processes and the effectiveness of your treatments.

So, both courses cover the same ground. There is however one notable difference. On the live course, your practical application is assessed. Practical assessment is not possible on the online course, but you have access to detailed video demonstrations of the appropriate technique for working each of the limbic reflex areas with the assessment component taking the form of a graded quiz.

How to use this book.

The text serves as the course book for both the in-person and online Limbic Reflexology Courses.

It has evolved from the live course and incorporates all the invaluable feedback from past students. The book's aim is for you to familiarise yourself with the nuclei and networks of the limbic brain.

The brain is extremely complex, and we cannot hope to gain any more than an overview of the processes involved. However, an insight into the principles involved will give you enough understanding to be able to make an educated assessment when you work the reflex areas and to formulate an interpretation of your findings.

For instance, in a chronic pain condition, you should be able to say that the problem is more likely to be associated with pain facilitator pathways or that of the descending analgesia pathway. Or you can say that there may be a problem in the regulation of the HPA or the Amygdala. With your background knowledge, you will know what areas to work to address these. In short, your treatments become more targeted and effective.

The book only discusses the nuclei whose corresponding reflex areas are currently identified in Limbic Reflexology.

The limbic reflex area maps show the reflex areas on the right hallux. The reflex areas on the left hallux are a mirror image of the right hallux.

The information about each nucleus briefly summarises the processes in which these nuclei are known or suspected to be involved in their regulation, and the problems that can arise when their function is compromised.

Often, when there is dysfunction in a process the problem arises through inefficient regulation. So, in addition to working the reflex areas for the nuclei known to be involved in any condition, you would also work the areas that help regulate them.

In the latter part of the book several conditions are discussed to briefly illustrate the role of the limbic networks in the condition.

The 'check your understanding' questions at the end of the book are designed to ensure you have understood the main points that will be of use in your practice. All the answers to the questions are to be found in the relevant section.

As a companion to this Course, I strongly recommend the 3D brain by Cold Spring Harbor Laboratories. This is available as an APP or it can be accessed on the 'Genes to Cognition Online' website.

This Course is a starting point. There is a goldmine of information available on the NCBI website. All the neuroscience in this book has been gleaned from such academic articles. I have not given any references here but links to the more accessible articles are on the Student Area of the Limbic website.

Limbic Reflexology view of the brain.

As I mentioned in the introduction, to accurately locate the limbic reflex areas on the foot the view of the brain is tilted back 45 degrees at the level of the midbrain. In the 3D Brain App this can be viewed so that the Amygdalae are at the same level as the Pituitary.

The face on, or coronal, view of the brain is found on the lateral half of the plantar hallux only. So, what about the medial half? The answer comes when we ask the question, 'Why do we work the Pituitary on both feet?'

There are two Amygdalae, two Hippocampi and two Striatum, but only one Pituitary.

Place the medial edge of your thumbs together with the Pituitary reflex areas touching each other.

The medial halves of the thumbs are in contact and where they are in contact, from medial edge to Pituitary, represents the midline of the brain.

Therefore, when you separate your thumbs, the medial half of the thumb corresponds to the profile view of the brain. Of course, this too is tilted, so you find reflex areas as illustrated below.

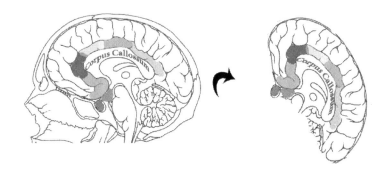

Limbic Reflexology view of the brain

So, in answer to our question, when we work the Pituitary reflex area on one foot, we are working half of the Pituitary and some of the Hypothalamus nuclei.

The Limbic Brain

(limbic = lining)

On the outside layer or shell of the brain is the cortex. Below the cortex are subcortical areas that include the limbic structures. Limbic means lining. So, the limbic brain lines the cortex.

As the primary role of the limbic brain is to detect and protect us from danger, it continually responds to danger signals in such a way as to maximise our chance of survival. It is highly regulated for optimum operation.

Because it has become so successful in doing this, it has withstood evolutionary selection and is well preserved in evolutionary terms. That means, because all vertebrate species have a limbic brain, it must pre-date the diversification of species. After diversification, some species evolved higher brain functions like our enlarged cortex or neocortex. In this sense, and only in this sense, the limbic brain is primitive.

The main role of the complex networks of the limbic brain is to continually monitor and respond to both the external and internal environments. In other words, what's going on around us, and what's happening inside our body.

An assessment of the significance of that information initiates an appropriate physiological, emotional, and behavioural response through the autonomic and endocrine nervous systems, in such a way as to optimise our survival and our adaptation to change. The limbic brain is where much of that processing takes place and where our responses are largely determined.

So, the limbic brain networks are at the centre of the regulatory processes that we call homeostasis, and it is the restoration of homeostatic norms that is at the centre of any reflexology treatment.

Central to its function, the limbic brain is the source of our primitive emotional responses like fear or anger. When limbic processes are dysregulated or disrupted, the result may be physiological imbalance or emotional disorder.

It is important to remember that the limbic brain should not be regarded as a separate entity. Rather, it is fully integrated with other areas of the brain and other body systems through complex connections and feedback processes.

This will become clearer when we explore memory, and the perception and control of pain. In addition, although our focus is the subcortical nuclei, some cortical areas have a limbic component and are closely associated with limbic functions.

Before we look at the individual nuclei, we need to get an overview of the landscape of the brain and its gross anatomy.

The Gross Structure of the Brain

Beneath the skull, there are three coverings of the brain and spinal cord called the meninges.

- The outside covering called the Dura Mater.
- The middle covering called the Arachnoid Mater.
- The covering clinging to the surface of the brain called the Pia Mater.

Between the Arachnoid and the Pia there is the sub-arachnoid space. This is filled with circulating cerebrospinal fluid (CSF).

CSF bathes the brain, supplying nutrients and removing waste products. It circulates around the brain, and is found in the subarachnoid space, four chambers or ventricles, their connecting aqueducts, and the spinal canal. In a lumbar puncture, CSF is collected from the subarachnoid space in the lower spine for analysis.

The Central Nervous System consists of the Brain and the Spinal Cord

The Cerebrum consists of:

- The Cortex – the outside layer, or shell, of the brain. This is the familiar convoluted covering of the brain, with its various lobes.
- Subcortical areas lie beneath the cortex and include the limbic structures. (Some areas of the of the cortex are also involved in limbic functions and are termed para-limbic.)

The Diencephalon is a subcortical structure. It lies above the brainstem. It consists of;

- The Thalamus.
- The Hypothalamus.
- The Epithalamus. (Between the posterior ends of the two Thalami, not shown in the diagram. The Epithalamus consists of the paired Habenula and the unpaired Pineal gland.)

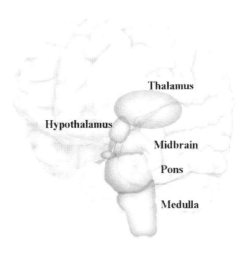

Below the Diencephalon is the Brainstem. The Brainstem consists of;

- The Midbrain.
- The Pons Varolli, or Pons.
- The Medulla Oblongata, or Medulla.

Behind the Pons is the Cerebellum, and below the brainstem and continuous with the brainstem is the spinal cord.

The Respiratory Centre and Cardiac Centre are found in the Medulla.

The Ascending Reticular Activating System (ARAS) in the brainstem influences our level of consciousness and the state of arousal.

Ten of the 12 pairs of cranial nerves have their nuclei in the brainstem. Cranial Nerves Three and Four have their nuclei in the Midbrain, Five to Eight in the Pons, and Nine to Twelve in the Medulla.

Cells of the Central Nervous System

Grey matter refers to the cell bodies of the brain tissue.

White matter refers to the fibres that transport information between cells. White matter is so called as most of the fibres are encased in a myelin sheath, which has a pale colour.

The cells of the brain, like other cells of the body, have a surrounding cell membrane, a central nucleus, and all the organelles in the cytoplasm that surrounds the nucleus.

Cells of the brain fall into three groups

- Glia cells.
- Microglia.
- Neurons.

Glia Cells got their name from the ancient idea that they functioned like glue holding everything together. We now know that they have much more complex functions in the physiology of the brain.

Astrocytes and Oligodendrocytes are two types of glia cells.

- Astrocytes are the most abundant cells in the brain. They perform many functions, including reabsorption of neurotransmitters around synapses, maintenance of neurons, building of synapses and as a structural scaffolding to prevent neurons becoming entangled. It is

7

thought that Astrocytes are involved in creating the Blood Brain Barrier.
- Oligodendrocytes form the myelin in myelinated fibres in the brain. (Schwann cells perform this function in the peripheral nervous system)

Microglia are involved in the immune response in the brain. However, they are much more than this. In the developing brain, they play a significant role in modelling the brain through processes such as pruning and natural cell death. Throughout life, they are crucial in the constantly remodelling that is involved in processes such as learning.

Neurons are the more familiar brain cell and are involved in signalling. They synthesise neurotransmitters and create action potentials or nerve impulses.

There are three main types of neurons:

- Motor neurons that carry signals from the brain to the tissues of the body.
- Sensory neurons carry signals from the tissues to the brain.
- Interneurons act as intermediate neurons that relay signals.

Afferent signals refer to information arriving at a cell.

Efferent signals are information that the cell sends out.

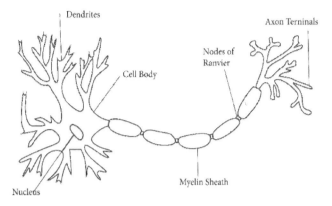

CNS Neuron

Neurons have:

- Dendrites. These receive signals from neighbouring cells.
- A cell body with a nucleus.
- Axons, which may or may not be, covered by a myelin sheath.
- Axon terminals. Action potentials, or nerve impulses, travel along the axon from the cell body to axon terminals at the end of the axon. In the axon terminals, there are vesicles containing neurotransmitters. Axon terminals form the interface with the dendrites of neighbouring neurons.

Some estimate, that there are over 1 trillion cells in the brain. Of that, there are only around 100 billion neurons. Each neuron fires between 5 and 50 times a second and can be in communication with 1000 other neurons at any one time.

Myelin Sheath.

Many, but not all, axons are sheathed in myelin. This is a fatty substance that insulates the axon and speeds up conduction of the signal.

In the Central Nervous System, myelin is formed by Oligodendrocytes and in the Peripheral Nervous System, Schwann cells form myelin.

Each Oligodendrocyte can insulate many fibres whereas each Schwann cell insulates only one, or part of one, peripheral fibre. Repair of myelin is much slower in the Central Nervous System (CNS) than in the Peripheral Nervous system (PNS).

Nodes of Ranvier are breaks in the myelin sheath where the nerve fibre is exposed. A nerve impulse can jump from node to node and so speed up the conduction of the impulse.

Action Potential (nerve impulse)

Neurons are irritable. That is, with excitatory stimulation, the cell body can generate an electrical impulse called an action potential. This action potential is conducted down the axon by chemical and electrical means towards the axon terminal. The impulse is transferred to the target cell across a connection called a synapse.

Chemical Synapse

There are several types of synapses, all working slightly differently. One type of synapse is a chemical synapse.

At chemical synapses, neurons do not touch each other.

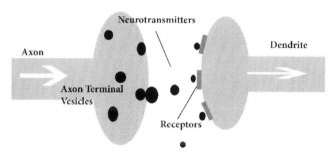

Diagram of a chemical synapse

Where the axon terminal of one neuron meets the dendrites of another there is a gap, or cleft, called the synaptic cleft. As mentioned above, at the axon terminal there are vesicles which store chemicals. These chemicals are called neurotransmitters. When the nerve impulse arrives, it triggers the release of these neurotransmitters into the synaptic cleft.

On the surface of the dendrites of the neighbouring neuron there are receptors protruding from the membrane. The neurotransmitters travel across the synaptic cleft and bind to these receptors. Depending on the nature of the neurotransmitter and the nature of the receptor, this can either excite or inhibit that cell. Where the effect is excitatory, then this will trigger an action potential or nerve impulse in the next neuron, and so the signal is passed on from neuron to neuron. If the effect is inhibitory, then it will prevent the signal passing on.

To affect a reaction from the receptors, the strength of the neurotransmitter signal must reach a certain level or threshold. We will meet up with this concept of threshold later.

One-to-one synapses are the exception. At a synapse, there may be thousands of axons influencing the same dendrite receptors and the membrane may be under the influence of both excitatory and inhibitory signals at the same time.

It is the overall sum or balance of these signals that determines whether the effect is inhibitory or excitatory.

There is a continuous process of excitatory and inhibitory signalling going on in the brain, and it is those excitatory and inhibitory events at synapses that underpin most of the activity and processes in the brain.

Not all the neurotransmitters are used up at the synapse. Excess neurotransmitters in the synaptic cleft are reabsorbed, in part by the action of Astrocytes, and recycled back into the axon terminal via transporters for further use.

Some drugs like SSRI antidepressants, target these transporters and inhibit reabsorption. SSRI antidepressants, like Fluoxetine, block the transporters that would normally reabsorb the excess Serotonin, (hence the name Selective Serotonin Reuptake Inhibitors). This increases the available Serotonin in the synapse hence prolonging its effect.

Amphetamine does the same thing for Dopamine.

In neuroendocrine neurons the chemicals released by the vesicles are released into the space between cells called the interstitial space, get absorbed into capillaries, and enter the circulation acting as hormones.

As an example of a neurohormone, Vasopressin, synthesised in the Hypothalamus, is released by axon terminal vesicles into the posterior Pituitary and enters directly into the bloodstream.

Receptors

There are hundreds of different receptors on the outside surface of a cell membrane. These are proteins spanning the membrane wall which control the opening and closing of channels in the cell membrane, thus controlling the flow of traffic across the membrane. This protects our cells from unwanted intruders whilst allowing raw materials that the cell needs to function, to cross the cell membrane.

Some receptors are sensitive to very specific signals. The receptor will only respond when a specific hormone or neurotransmitter binds with it.

Others may be sensitive to more than one neurotransmitter or have a greater affinity, or respond more, to one neurotransmitter than another.

Other receptors require a cofactor such as magnesium, in addition to the neurotransmitter or hormone, before it is activated.

Not only does a receptor require a signal to become activated, its activation also depends on the strength of that signal. Only when the signal strength reaches this level, or threshold, will it be triggered. When a receptor is activated, the membrane is said to have become depolarised.

As a normal function of homeostasis, the number and sensitivity of receptors constantly vary. Changes in the number of receptors and the sensitivity of receptors at synapses underlie the phenomenon of learning.

However, in many conditions the disruption of homeostasis can be caused by, or results in, abnormal changes in the density or sensitivity of receptors. This is the case in many chronic pain conditions where there may be Central Nervous System sensitisation with chronically oversensitive receptors.

Many, if not most, medicines and toxins have their effect on receptors either modifying them by making them sensitive, or blocking them, as is the case with anaesthetics or snake venom.

Neurotransmitters

When protein in our diet is digested, the protein is eventually broken down to amino acids. In our body, there are 20 such amino acids.

These 20 amino acids become the building blocks, or raw material, that are used to make, or synthesise, all the proteins that the body needs. DNA is the recipe book for making those proteins. The amino acids are assembled in the cells one by one according to the recipe.

A long chain of amino acids is assembled and then folded over to form the new protein. The order, sequence of assembly, and the folding will determine which protein is made. All the protein recipes are synthesised from those 20 amino acids ingredients, each protein having their individual order of assembly according to the DNA recipe.

A neurotransmitter is just one of those synthesised proteins derived from amino acids.

For example, Dopamine is derived from the amino acid Tyrosine. In the brain, Tyrosine is modified in steps to produce L-Tyrosine, L-Dopa and then Dopamine.

Dopamine is further modified to synthesise Norepinephrine, which in turn is modified to produce Epinephrine.

(Tyrosine is also the base amino acid in the synthesis of Thyroxine. Tyrosine, with three or four iodine molecules attached, gives us T3 and T4 respectively.)

Serotonin is derived from the amino acid Tryptophan. Melatonin is modified Serotonin.

The Blood Brain Barrier is a collection of endothelial cells, Astrocytes and microglia with tight gap junctions between them. The BBB separates the circulating blood from the extracellular fluid of the brain. This barrier allows free passage of nutrients and oxygen needed by the brain, whilst denying access to foreign material that may be harmful to the brain.

One of the criteria in this filter process is the size of molecule and neurotransmitter molecules are simply too big to get through. So, where there is a deficiency of these chemicals, we cannot simply ingest supplements.

For example, in Parkinson's Disease, we cannot take Dopamine supplement to increase depleted Dopamine levels. However, L-Dopa molecules can cross the blood brain barrier. L-Dopa can then be modified in the brain to synthesise Dopamine.

You will find that your client suffering from Parkinson's Disease will most likely be prescribed medication containing L-Dopa.

Common Neurotransmitters in the CNS

Neurotransmitters can be excitatory or inhibitory. At its simplest, all neural processes involve a series of excitatory and inhibitory events.

Glutamate is an excitatory neurotransmitter. (Glutamate is one of the essential amino acids.)

Gamma aminobutyric acid (GABA) is the main inhibitory neurotransmitter in the brain.

Drugs designed to calm brain activity target GABA receptors. For example, benzodiazepines like Diazepam, antiepileptic medications like Gabapentin, (often used as an analgesic) all enhance the inhibitory effect of GABA receptors.

Dopamine is widespread in the brain. Dis-regulation of Dopamine levels is implicated in conditions such as Depression and Parkinson's Disease, whilst excess Dopamine may be a factor in Schizophrenia.

Some drugs of misuse, like amphetamines, and cocaine, have their effect by increasing the dopamine levels in the brain.

Norepinephrine is a common neurotransmitter in arousal circuits. It is also involved in sleep wake cycles, maintenance of muscle tone, and, as we shall see, pain inhibitory and facilitation pathways.

Serotonin is implicated in mood disorders and in pain inhibition. Only 20% of the body's Serotonin is found in the brain. Most Serotonin is found in the gut where it is involved in peristalsis. It is also the neurotransmitter involved in the initiation of breathing.

Like Dopamine, ingested Serotonin is unable to cross the blood brain barrier. Eating Serotonin-rich foods, like nettles, is more likely to alter your bowel habits rather than your mood.

The Limbic Brain Nuclei and Reflex Areas

Nuclei are a group of cells being in close proximity, have similar structure and are observed to have some common function. There are countless nuclei in the limbic brain. Here we explore those for which we have a corresponding reflex area.

Limbic reflex areas are precision areas. At the time of writing, there are around 30 discreet limbic reflex areas.

We are already familiar with three of them: The Pituitary, Adrenals and spinal reflex T9. The Pituitary reflex area appears all the maps to serve as a point of reference.

Doubtless to say, more reflex areas may be identified in time to come, but for now, we will explore only those that have a corresponding limbic reflex area.

Working techniques in Limbic Reflexology are an adaptation of some of the techniques we already use with a few additional techniques.

- Walking.
- Rolling with the thumb.
- Hook.
- Resting.

These are depicted on the reflex maps by W, R, H and Re.

The holding hand as always, provides the stability for working the reflex areas. The fingers of the working hand provide fine control in applying the techniques, just as resting the heel of the hand provides fine control when we write.

Pressure and speed of working are crucial in Limbic Reflexology. The limbic reflex areas are precision areas, and slow even pressure is crucial in detecting the reflex areas.

Pressure needs to be even and controlled. To avoid thumb fatigue and strain, pressure and variation in pressure is controlled by both the holding hand and the fingers of the working hand.

Areas of contact on the working thumb.

We are used to employing the 'corner' point of the thumb in working reflex areas. In Limbic Reflexology we use both 'corners' and for the roll technique, the fleshy thumb between those two corners. With practice, this area of the thumb will become finely tuned in detecting the nuances of the reflex areas.

Insula or Insular Cortex

The Insula lies deep within the fold between the parietal, and temporal lobes. If we could peel the temporal lobe outwards, we would expose the Insular Cortex in the parietal lobe. The Insula is shaped like an open fan. It spans an area from the orbitofrontal to the sensory parietal.

The Insula is often seen as three units in one, with posterior, middle, and anterior parts. The mid-Insula is not fully understood, but is thought in part, to be involved in sensory awareness, or interoception.

As it is difficult to detect a distinct mid-insular reflex area, for our purposes, we will identify two areas – posterior, and anterior.

The Anterior Insula (AI), is functionally distinct from the Posterior Insula (PI). The Posterior Insula is thought to be one of the areas where sensory information from the body arrives via the Thalamus. So, the posterior Insula is involved primarily with interoceptive awareness – what's going on in the body.

The function of the Insula gradually changes towards the anterior end where it is more involved in evaluating information and in initiating appropriate emotional responses based on the survival salience (significance) of this information. Information interpreted as a threat to homeostasis or survival, demands priority attention.

The Insula has been extensively investigated and a whole host of functions has been attributed to it. Some of these are listed here.

- Part of the Salience Network (salience = how significant an event is) The Saliency Network is discussed below.
- Interoceptive awareness, that is, an awareness of all our internal body states. Timing of the heartbeat, blood pressure etc.
- Maps visceral states associated with emotional experience.
- Sensation of intensity of pain. Emotional response to pain.
- Awareness of warm/cold. Awareness of stomach or bladder distension.
- Regulation of the sympathetic NS.
- Regulation of the immune system.
- Involved in the sense of self (me/not me). Sense of body ownership (what I can feel, and sense is only truly known to me).
- Involved in empathy. Imagines pain, when observing others pain or pictures of suffering. On MRI scans, imagined pain activates the same areas as would, actual pain.
- Role in motor recovery from stroke.
- Sense of disgust e.g. noxious smells.
- Norm violations.

In major Depression and in chronic pain conditions, there are structural and functional abnormalities, which may lead to altered information processing of interoceptive signals, with exaggerated responses.

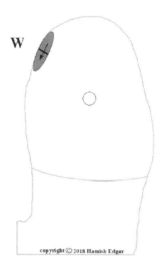

Insula Reflex Area

When we are working the Insula reflex area in pain conditions, it is useful to note differences in tenderness and texture between the AI and PI. The PI would tell us more about the perceived intensity of pain, and the AI would inform us more about the emotional response.

Amygdala

There are two Amygdalae. These are almond-shaped groups of nuclei located deep within each of the medial temporal lobes of the cerebrum. (Amygdala means almond in Latin)

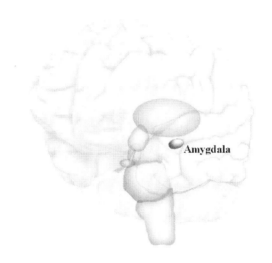

The amygdalae receive and send information to and from many areas of the brain and are involved in many processes.

- Activation of the Amygdala is an involuntary and unconscious process.
- Not activated in conscious emotional responses.
- Detects significant emotional arousal, both positive and negative.

- Better known for emergency responses to negative situations.
- It is involved in encoding, storage, and retrieval of episodic-autobiographical memory (EAM), that is, events, or experience.
- Amygdala checks the context of sensory signals against its memory bank.
- Arousal is dependent on the strength of the memory for the event.
- Memories of an emotional event elicit an unconscious neurological and endocrinal response.
- Involved in the origin of many fear responses including freezing (immobility) and startle response.
- Involved in the initiation of a cascade of physiological responses that results in the fight or flight response.
- Processes reactions to violations concerning personal space.
- It is dimorphic, that is, like many of the brain's structures, there are differences between female and male Amygdalae.
- It is regulated to some extent by the prefrontal cortex and is reciprocally regulated by the Hippocampus. (see below)
- Involved in endogenous pain control i.e. the body's own control of pain.

The Amygdala has been associated with a several disorders:

- Depressed patients show exaggerated left Amygdala activity.
- In PTSD, the Amygdalae are enlarged and overactive.
- In chronic pain conditions, Amygdala function is impaired.
- The left Amygdala is hyperactive in Bipolar Depression. People with Bipolar Disorder tend to have considerably smaller Amygdalae.
- Connections between the Amygdala and Autism.
- Link between the Amygdala and schizophrenia - the right Amygdala is significantly larger than the left.

The Basolateral Nucleus (BLA) of the Amygdala activates another area of the Amygdala, the Central Nucleus (CE). It does this via interneurons called Intercalated Cells (ITC) which are located at the interface of the BLA and CE. These ITC cells are regulated by the infralimbic prefrontal cortex which is discussed below.

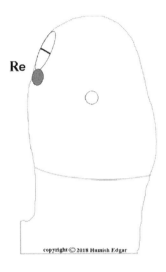

Re

Amygdala Reflex Area

Hippocampus.

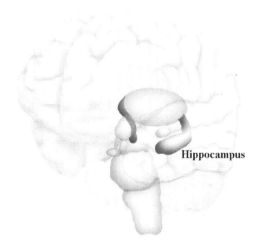

The Hippocampus is situated in the temporal lobe and extends backwards curving over to the mammillary bodies below the Hypothalamus. It is mainly involved in learning and memory. The Hippocampus gives us a spatial map and is concerned with the context of memories.

It creates an association between a memory and a specific place or situation. This gives us a familiarity with our environment. The Hippocampus is pivotal in learning.

The internal structure of the Hippocampus is difficult to envisage. Think of it as a rolled-up newspaper, rolled up one way, then rolled back on itself. In early times, the cross-section view of the Hippocampus was thought to resemble a sea horse, hence the name which in Greek, means 'sea horse'.

- Major role in learning and memory.
- Regulates Hypothalamus-Pituitary-Adrenal axis (HPA) (see Subiculum below).
- The Amygdala and Hippocampus regulate each other.
- The Hippocampus is very much involved in the neurobiology of Depression.
- In Alzheimer's Disease, this area is often one of the first to be affected.

Hippocampus formation

Various sub-structures make up the Hippocampal Formation. Each has been accredited with specific functions.

One specific area, the Fusiform Gyrus, is involved in the recognition of fearful faces whilst another part of the formation is the Dentate Gyrus, the site where neurogenesis was first detected.

Research into Depression has indicated atrophy in the Hippocampus. The Hippocampus is rich in Glucocorticoid Receptors (GR), the target receptors of Cortisol.

In chronic stress, continuous high Cortisol levels can overexcite these receptors and damage dendrites in the Hippocampus resulting in atrophy and loss of connections.

Stress also activates cytokines - pro-inflammatory agents of the immune system in the brain. Again, the Hippocampus is very sensitive to cytokines.

For those with a history of early life trauma, this may alter the development of the Hippocampus. It will still develop, but in a way that will bestow a vulnerability to mental health issues, including Anxiety and Depression.

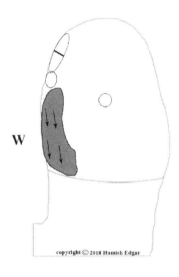

Hippocampus Reflex Area

Subiculum.

One of the areas of the Hippocampus that we are interested in is the Subiculum. The Subiculum is the main outlet for signals from the Hippocampus and our interest lies in its role in the regulation of the HPA axis. In many conditions, such as Depression, this regulatory control of the HPA is compromised resulting in a hyperactive HPA Axis.

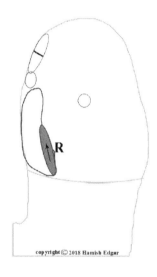

Subiculum Reflex Area

Locus Coeruleus

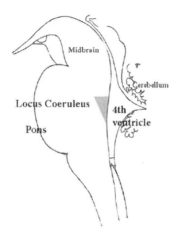

Location of the Locus Coeruleus

locus= spot, or location, coeruleus= blue (Cerulean blue, is familiar to artists)

The Locus Coeruleus (LC) is a nucleus at the back of the Pons in the brainstem. It is the main, almost exclusive, source of Norepinephrine (Noradrenaline) in the brain.

- Norepinephrine in the brain acts as an excitatory neurotransmitter and is involved in many arousal systems in the brain.
- The Locus Coeruleus is a major player in stress and any condition where heightened arousal is a major feature.

- The LC innervates the forebrain initiating the cognitive response to stress, that is the thinking component to stress
- In stress, it influences bowel motility.
- Influences the endocrine functions via its influence on the Hypothalamus and the peripheral autonomic nervous system.
- Involved in circadian rhythms due to its role in arousal levels.
- Involved in memory consolidation and extinction.
- Plays a major role in the perception of pain and in pain inhibition.

The Locus Coeruleus neurons have two different modes of firing: a phasic mode, and tonic mode. When we are focussing on a task, it fires in the slower phasic mode. It switches to the tonic mode when we are scanning our environment or deciding our response options to sensory information. So, the mode will be the one that will set the most appropriate level of arousal to deal with incoming information.

In stress, there is heightened arousal due to CRH stimulation of the Locus Coeruleus by the Amygdala and Hypothalamus.

During sleep, the Locus Coeruleus is largely inactive.

Like many areas of the brain, the LC is dimorphic, that is, it is different in males and females. In females, there are more CRH receptors, more dendrites, (more connections), and those dendrites extend further than in males. It has been suggested that this may partly explain why females are more prone to anxiety disorders.

Dysfunction of the Locus Coeruleus has been implicated in several conditions:

- Stress, Anxiety, and panic attack
- Parkinson's Disease, where there is loss of Locus Coeruleus neurons.
- Pain Control, especially Neuropathic pain.
- Alzheimer's Disease.
- OCD, where anxiety is a major feature.
- Depression.
- Post-Traumatic Stress Disorder (PTSD).

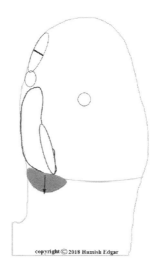

Locus Coeruleus Reflex Area

Thalamus.

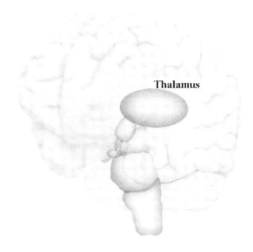

Thalamus

There are two Thalami. Each Thalamus is situated either side of the third ventricle and joined by a stalk like a dumbbell that passes though the ventricle.

There are numerous subdivisions of the Thalamus, each accredited with differing functions. For our purposes, we will divide it into posterior, at the bottom of the reflex area, mid, and anterior areas.

The Thalamus is the main relay station for afferent (incoming) information from the spinal cord and from other brain areas.

The Thalamus however is not simply a passive sorting office. Each piece of information is subject to change and influence from other signals during its transit through the Thalamus.

Each distinct area of the Thalamus receives and relays information to different parts of the brain. These have been grouped into pathways. Our main interest is in what is termed the Medial Pathway.

The Medial Pathway

The Medial Pathway projects from the Thalamus to subcortical areas with which we are already familiar. These include the Insula, Cingulate, Amygdala, Hippocampus and the basal ganglia, (which includes the Substantia Nigra and Striatum.)

Often you can distinguish differing textures in each part of the Thalamus reflex area.

Posterior Thalamus
Often tender in IBS allergic conditions and Asthma. Involved in pain signal relay from the spinal cord.

Mid-Thalamus
Invariably tender in pain and chronic pain, where it is sensitised to pain.

Anterior Thalamus
Involved in cognitive and emotional responses and memory. Projects heavily to limbic structures.

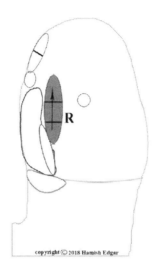

Thalamus Reflex Area

Striatum.

The Striatum is the collective name for the Caudate and the Putamen and is part of a group of areas known collectively as the Basal Ganglia.

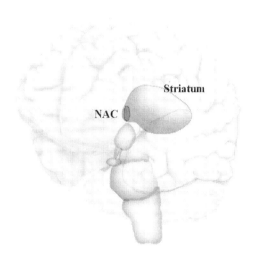

The Striatum is well connected to limbic structures, including the Amygdala, Hippocampus, Prefrontal Cortex (PFC), brainstem nuclei and Cingulate Cortex.

- The Striatum is involved in initiating and fine-tuning voluntary movements. It depends on a supply of Dopamine from the midbrain.
- The Striatum is involved in memory, contributing to learning, habitual behaviours, and performance of tasks.
- It is involved in behavioural flexibility and in inhibiting behaviours in complex social interactions.
- Involved in OCD and ADHD.

In Parkinson's Disease, the Striatum receives insufficient Dopamine supply from the Substantia Nigra in the midbrain, which impairs the ability of the Striatum to orchestrate the control of fine movements.

As well as its involvement in Parkinson's Disease, impairment of striatal functioning is also the focus of the problems in Huntington's Disease. This is not due to inadequate Dopamine but is a genetic disease where a mutant gene produces a protein that destroys neurons. The first place this occurs is in the Striatum.

In OCD, it is thought that there are altered connections between the Anterior Cingulate Cortex, Prefrontal Cortex, and the Striatum.

Nucleus Accumbens.

Often referred to as the Ventral Striatum, the Nucleus Accumbens (NAc) is involved in seeking rewards and thus is a major player in learning and motivation. If there is expected reward from a given set of behaviours, then the Nucleus Accumbens and Striatum will orchestrate the actions required to get that reward, or if the outcome is undesirable then they will initiate action to avoid it.

- The NAc has a role in initiating behaviours towards goals, and rewards.
- Ascertains if behaviour is proceeding towards desired goals.
- Has two modes – approach/seeking, towards desirable goals and aversion/avoidance with undesirable outcomes.
- In some conditions, such as Depression, can get 'stuck' in aversion/avoidance mode.
- Relies on Dopamine from the VTA in the midbrain.
- Sometimes referred to as the 'pleasure centre'.
- Significant player in addiction. Drugs like cocaine and amphetamines increase the available Dopamine in the Nucleus Accumbens.
- The reward circuit includes the NAc, Cingulate, and Orbitofrontal Cortex (discussed later).
- Dysfunction of the Nucleus Accumbens is implicated in Obsessive Compulsive Disorder (OCD) .
- Dysfunctional reward circuits are also implicated in Depression, where there is lowered

motivation, apathy, and loss of pleasure (anhedonia).

Striatum & Nucleus Accumbens
Reflex areas

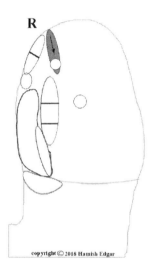

Orbitofrontal Cortex

The Orbitofrontal Cortex (OFC) is part of the prefrontal Cortex, often referred to as the lateral prefrontal cortex and is anatomically continuous with the anterior Insula.

- Involved in calculating the expected value or cost of potential outcomes of competing options.
- Relays this to the Prefrontal Cortex, Cingulate, and NAc. which influences decision making, learning, and behaviour.
- OFC has substantial anatomical connections with the Amygdala.
- Important in anxiety states where there are heightened expectancies of threat.
- Thought to be dysfunctional in chronic low back pain.
- It is thought that the OFC may help regulate the reward circuit.
- Part of the Default Mode Network.

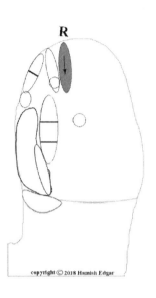

R

Orbitofrontal Cortex Reflex Area

Subgenual Anterior Cingulate

The Corpus Callosum is the broad band of fibres that exchange signals between the two hemispheres of the brain.

The Cingulate Cortex is a narrow 'collar' of cortex that lies along the top of the Corpus Callosum.

The Cingulate bends under the Callosum at its anterior end. This bend is called the genu (knee) and the part of below the knee is the Subgenual Anterior Cingulate, or sgACC. The part on or around the bend or genu is termed the perigenual ACC, or pgACC.

We can divide the sgACC into anterior and posterior parts, the posterior part being at the end of the 'collar'. Both parts of the sgACC have strong connections to limbic areas.

The anterior sgACC is mainly involved in attention and emotion processing. (Also, in recall of memory and fear memory extinction). The anterior sgACC corresponds to the top half of the reflex area.

The posterior sgACC, the bottom half of the reflex area, is thought to be homogeneous to an area of the Prefrontal Cortex called the Infralimbic PFC, and for our purposes we will regard it as such. This is involved in the regulation of the Amygdala.

Connections from this infralimbic area regulate the flow of information between two parts of the Amygdala, the Basolateral and the Central Amygdala Complex. In some conditions like PTSD and OCD, this regulation by the infralimbic cortex is impaired. Continuous and accumulating sleep debt that can be experienced in everyday life can also downregulate this suppression of the Amygdala by the sgACC.

Often when the Amygdala is tender, the problem is one of regulation. Working the posterior sgACC reflex area often results in a reduction of any Amygdala tenderness.

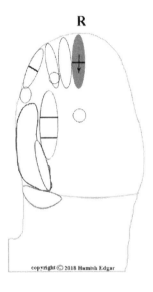

Subgenual ACC Reflex Area

Pituitary

The Pituitary gland, often referred to as the master gland, is situated in the hypophyseal fossa of the sphenoid bone at the level of the bridge of our nose. It is connected to the Hypothalamus by a stalk.

- Part of the Hypothalamus-Pituitary-Adrenal Axis (discussed below)
- Hormonal regulation
- Production of endorphins

The Anterior and Posterior Pituitary have differing embryonic origins. The Anterior Pituitary originates from the roof of the embryonic mouth cavity and herniates upwards. The Posterior Pituitary started life as part of the Hypothalamus which herniated down so that the Anterior and Posterior Pituitary come together.

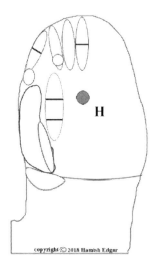

Pituitary Reflex Area

Hypothalamus

The Hypothalamus is situated below the Thalamus, hence hypo-thalamus, and behind and above the Pituitary, and that is where we find the reflex area. It consists of around 12 groups of nuclei, situated within the walls of the third ventricle

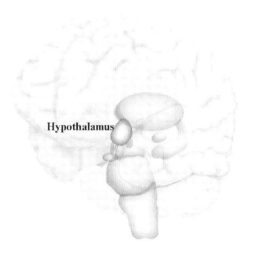

Location of the Hypothalamus

The Hypothalamus is by far the most influential limbic area in maintaining homeostasis. Other limbic nuclei all compete to influence the Hypothalamus either directly or indirectly, and the Hypothalamus is the main output of limbic processes.

The Hypothalamus has countless connections and Its nuclei are involved in a wide range of the body's homeostatic processes. These include:

- Regulation of the endocrine system.
- Control of fertility.
- Control, and regulation of, ovarian cycles. The Hypothalamus is the target of contraceptive medication.
- Control of the Autonomic Nervous System.
- Control of the Reproductive System.
- Control of circadian cycles, and the Pineal Gland.
- Control of the Pituitary Gland.
- Regulation of emotional states.
- Regulation of eating, and drinking.
- Control of body temperature.
- Part of the Hypothalamus-Pituitary-Adrenal Axis.

The Hypothalamus secretes at least nine known hormones, all of them trophic, that is they target other endocrine glands.

The Hypothalamus produces both releasing and inhibitory hormones. Most Hypothalamic hormones travel down the Pituitary stalk and enter the Anterior Pituitary via a portal blood system. Once in the Anterior Pituitary, they stimulate or inhibit the production and release of Pituitary hormones.

Each hormone is regulated by negative feedback loops. Receptors in the Hypothalamus monitor hormone levels in the blood and either secrete a releasing hormone to increase the level of the hormone or if levels are adequate or high, an inhibiting hormone to stop the production of the Anterior Pituitary hormone.

Neuroendocrine neurons secrete hormones directly into the Posterior Pituitary. Vasopressin and Oxytocin are hormones synthesised in the Hypothalamus and released from the terminal vesicles into the Posterior Pituitary.

It may be useful to think of the nuclei of the Hypothalamus as resembling a bunch of grapes, with the stalk pointing towards the Pituitary. In a coronal view, face on, it is seen that the nuclei are arranged in three vertical zones either side of the midline.

We are particularly interested in six of the nuclei clusters.

- Paraventricular Nucleus (PVN)
- Preoptic Nucleus (PO)
- Lateral Nucleus (LHA)
- Tuberomammillary Nucleus (TMN)
- Suprachiasmic Nucleus (SCN)
- Mammillary Bodies (MB)

Paraventricular Nucleus (PVN)

Found in the central zone, the PVN produces the hormones TRH, CRH, PRH, Oxytocin and Somatostatin. The Paraventricular nucleus also measures circulating Cortisol and so is involved in the feedback loop regulating the HPA which we will be discussing later.

In the Middle Zones, either side of the central zone, we find the Preoptic Nucleus, the Suprachiasmatic Nucleus (SCN) and the Mammillary Bodies.

Preoptic Nucleus (PO)

The Preoptic Nucleus is involved in sleep/wake cycles and produces gonadotrophic hormone and LHRH.

It is also involved in thermoregulation. The cells involved in thermoregulation are activated by histamine from the TMN.

Lateral Hypothalamus Nucleus (LHA)

Found in the lateral zone, the Lateral Hypothalamus is involved in the regulation of arousal, motivation to feed, energy balance, stress, reward and motivated behaviour. The LHA is also involved in autonomic functions including heart rate, thermogenesis and energy storage.

Two of the LHA cell types are neurons that express Orexins, and Melanin Concentrating Hormone (MCH).

Orexin (OX) is also known as Hypocretin. It was discovered in 1998 by two separate groups at the same time and each gave it a different name.

- Orexin is involved in diverse processes including arousal, feeding behaviours, learning and autonomic functions involving the cardiac, respiratory and gastrointestinal systems.
- Orexin promotes wakefulness. Orexin influences the sleep wake transition and loss of Orexin underpins the problems found in Narcolepsy.
- Orexin is inhibited by the inflammatory response – animals sleep when ill.
- Orexin is reduced with age with increased sleepiness and lowered motivation for activity.
- Orexin promotes the arousal and the motivation to seek food. Leptin is an indicator of energy storage. Leptin is produced by adipose tissue in direct proportion to the amount of body fat. Normally, an increase in Leptin levels affect the LHA by suppressing Orexin and thus the motivation to seek food. Where Leptin resistance

develops, feeding behaviours are not inhibited which can lead to obesity.

Melanin Concentrating Hormone (MCH).

- MCH is sleep promoting and promotes REM sleep.
- It is involved in the control of energy expenditure and helps regulate white and brown adipose tissue.
- Influences energy saving during sleep (heart rate and motor activity).
- Implicated in regulating anxiety.
- Regulates intestinal tone.

Tuberomammillary Nucleus (TMN)

The TMN is found towards the base of the Hypothalamus. It produces histamine. As already mentioned, it influences thermoregulation by activating cells in the Preoptic Nucleus.

TMN promotes wakefulness by inhibiting MCH in the Lateral Hypothalamus, which helps explain why some Antihistamine medication induces drowsiness.

Suprachiasmatic Nucleus (SCN)

The Suprachiasmatic Nuclei are found above the optic chiasma where the optic nerves cross over just in front of the Hypothalamus and above the Pituitary. The nuclei serve as the body's 'master clock' to which all other 'clocks' in the body, are set.

The SCN receives signals from the retina. This includes information regarding the level of light entering the eye. This triggers a chain of events which results in a variation in the level of Norepinephrine at the Pineal Gland. It is this level of Norepinephrine to which the Pineal responds

When we work the Pituitary reflex area, we assume we are also working the Pineal reflex area. However, the Pineal gland is part of the Epithalamus and is found towards the back of the Thalamus, below the level of the Pituitary. Any beneficial effect on sleep through working the Pituitary is more likely to be due to the proximity of the SCN reflex area rather than the Pineal. The Suprachiasmatic Reflex area is found at 11 o'clock on the right foot, and 1 o'clock on the left in relation to the Pituitary reflex area. It is a precision area and feels like a pinhead.

Include the SCN in your treatment for any condition involving circadian cycles, including sleep, cortisol levels and reproductive cycle problems.

Mammillary Bodies(MB)

The Mammillary Bodies lie below the main body of the Hypothalamus. It is thought that they are involved in memory, acting as a relay between the Hippocampus and the anterior Thalamus.

At post mortem, the Mammillary Bodies are atrophied in those with alcoholic dementia, Korsakoff's Syndrome, where prolonged alcohol misuse leads to thiamine deficiency which results in memory impairment.

The Mammillary Body Reflex area is found at 7 o'clock on the right foot and 5 o'clock on the left in relation to the Pituitary reflex area. They are easier to detect than the SCN.

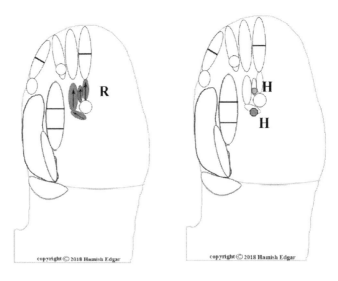

Hypothalamus Reflex Areas   SCN & MB Reflex Areas

Midline Hypothalamus

The midline Hypothalamus nuclei are found on the medial side of the toe which as we have seen represent the profile view of the brain.

Gender differences of the Hypothalamus

A surge of testosterone in the first few months after birth, sexualises the Hypothalamus. This results in a different distribution of oestrogen receptors and differences in functions of some of the Hypothalamic Nuclei.

- The pattern of secretion of growth hormone is different – males grow more.
- The Preoptic nucleus is much larger in males
- The Suprachiasmatic Nucleus (SCN) is larger in homosexual males.
- The sexualisation of the Hypothalamus determines the preferred attraction to pheromones – males are attracted to oestrogen, and females to testosterone.

We will be returning to the Hypothalamus when we explore the process that is central to the stress response, and homeostasis - the Hypothalamus-Pituitary-Adrenal Axis.

Bed Nucleus of the Stria Terminalis (BNST)

The BNST is part of what is referred to as the extended Amygdala.

The Stria Terminalis is a white matter bundle from the amygdala, that wraps around the Thalamus, and descends to the Bed Nucleus of the Stria Terminalis, above and forward from the Hypothalamus. There are extensive connections between the BNST and other limbic regions.

These limbic connections of the BNST form an anxiety circuit.

- Whilst the Amygdala becomes active when faced with predictable and immediate threat the BNST is activated by unpredictable threat.
- Increased activation of the BNST is present in hypervigilance typical of PTSD, and in situations where the potential for threat in uncertain and unpredictable and where the threat is habitually overestimated.
- the BNST is composed of several sub-nuclei and they regulate anxiety in opposite directions. Some increase anxiety whilst others decreases anxiety.
- We know the sgACC helps regulate the Amygdala. In addition, the Subgenual cingulate also influences the BNST.
- The Amygdala and the BNST project to the Hypothalamus and to brain stem areas which

modulate various features of anxiety such as heart rate and respiratory rate. Activity in the BNST influences the stress response of the HPA.

- So, the sgACC, the Hippocampus, the Amygdala and BNST, constitute a network which when coordinated controls and regulates anxiety.
- BNST neurons inhibit the lateral Hypothalamus which can result in increased eating behaviours. This may help explain in the weight gain and abnormal eating behaviours in anxiety disorders.
- A lot of research also suggests that the BNST is involved in the stress-induced reinstatement of drug seeking. This research points to the high incidence of trait anxiety and drug addiction.

We are particularly interested in this circuit when we have a client who has a problem with long term or sustained anxiety. When there is imbalance within the BNST between the anxiety promoting and anxiety inhibition processes, or there is ineffective regulation, this may result in sustained anxiety.

So, the BNST reflex area would be a cornerstone of our treatment plan for problems of chronic or sustained anxiety including Post Trauma Stress.

We will be looking at Anxiety and PTS later in this book.

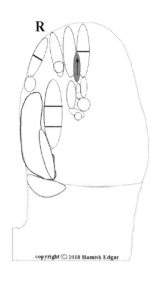

R

BNST Reflex Area

Periaqueductal Grey (PAG)

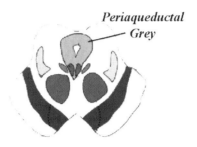

Periaqueductal Grey

Diagram of a section of the midbrain showing the PAG. The two black bars are the Substantia Nigra, and the two circular areas are the red nucleus.

The tube carrying cerebrospinal fluid through the midbrain, connecting the third and fourth ventricles, is called the aqueduct. The Periaqueductal Grey (PAG), or Central Grey, refers to a group of nuclei surrounding this aqueduct, hence Peri-aqueductal.

The PAG runs centrally from just below the Pituitary, to the level of the Locus Coeruleus.

- The PAG is best known for its involvement in the body's pain inhibitory pathways and in the descending analgesia pathway. It is rich in opioid receptors.
- It is also involved in the sympathetic response to stress, the panic response and the startle response.
- Involved in fear and fear memory.

- It is thought that the PAG is involved in the visceral response to emotional stress. It initiates the increased heart rate, blood pressure, and respiratory rate in response to stress.
- Dysfunction of PAG is thought to be involved in the complex pattern of migraine attacks.
- It sends and receives projections to many other brain areas including the Amygdala and the Cingulate.

Raphe Nucleus.

The Raphe Nucleus is a large group of nuclei, running through the brainstem.

- Produces the brain's Serotonin.
- In the descending analgesia pathway (discussed later) the PAG projects to the Raphe to stimulate Serotonin production. This Serotonin has the effect of dampening down pain processes at the level of the spinal cord.
- Serotonin is also a major neurotransmitter in the forebrain in cognitive and emotional processes
- Involved in respiration. The Respiratory Centre relies on Serotonin to initiate inspiration.

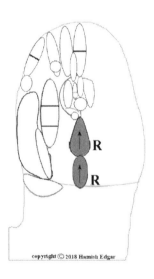

Periaqueductal Grey and Raphe Reflex Areas

Substantia Nigra / VTA

The Substantia Nigra, part of the Basal Ganglia, is a group of nuclei in the midbrain that release Dopamine. The 'Nigra' refers to the dark melanin pigment formed from the metabolic breakdown of Dopamine. Both the Striatum and Nucleus Accumbens rely on Dopamine supply.

Poor supply of Dopamine to the Striatum is the underlying problem in Parkinson's Disease.

The Substantia Nigra is also found to be dysfunctional and enlarged in ADHD.

Nearby in the midbrain is an area called the Ventral Tegmental Area (VTA) which also produces Dopamine. The Dopamine in the NAc originates in the VTA. Signalling to and from the VTA is involved in numerous processes.

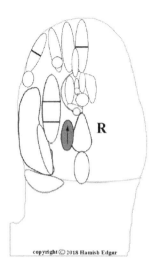

Substantia Nigra and VTA Reflex Area

Cingulate Cortex

The Cingulate is involved in determining what information gets attention and in selecting appropriate responses. It is also involved in error detection which means it detects if an outcome is what we intended from our actions, and initiates adjustments to our responses in light of that.

The Cingulate acts as the crossroads between emotion and thinking and thus integrates emotional and cognitive information.

The information below is complex but well worth learning. We have reflex areas that distinguish the various areas of the Cingulate and the Cingulate is involved in many of the conditions we encounter.

The Cingulate Cortex can be divided into several main sections.

- The Posterior Cingulate Cortex (PCC).
- The Mid-Cingulate (MCC).
- The Anterior Cingulate Cortex (ACC).
- The Subgenual Cingulate (sgACC) which we have already encountered.

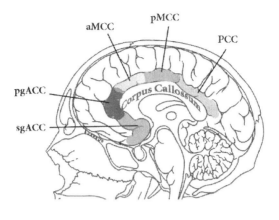

Cingulate Cortex

Posterior Cingulate Cortex (PCC)

The PCC is thought to be involved in generating autonomic responses and is active in retrieving autobiographical memories.

The PCC is one of the main areas involved in the Default Mode Network, the mode activated when we are engaged in internal thoughts and ruminations. When we switch to task activated thinking the PCC is less activated.

Ritalin, prescribed in ADHD, is thought to have its main influence in the PCC.

Although the Insular Cortex, the Anterior Cingulate Cortex and the PFC, are cortical structures, they all have a strong limbic function and extensive limbic connections.

Mid-Cingulate Cortex (MCC)

The MCC has two parts; the anterior and posterior MCC, (aMCC and pMCC)

The MCC is involved in reward related activity in conjunction with the Nucleus Accumbens, and is also involved in error detection, which is an integral part of learning and focused problem solving.

In OCD, it is thought that this error detection function is compromised. Dysfunctional error detection creates the sense that something is 'not quite right' or completed.

The MCC, in conjunction with the OFC, is involved in the selection of responses and the reward value of options. Its function is mainly cognitive (thinking) in nature.

The MCC is also involved in processing emotional responses and is involved in the acquisition of fear and the context of fear.

Anterior Mid-Cingulate Cortex (aMCC)

The aMCC gets information from all sections of the Cingulate and devises an action plan by way of an appropriate response.

This area is involved in the subjective rating of the unpleasantness, or the suffering component, of pain. (The Insula, as we have seen, is involved in rating the intensity of pain).

There is an area in the aMCC called the Rostral Cingulate Zone (RCZ). The functions of emotions, pain, and cognition are thought to overlap in the RCZ. It has many connections to limbic areas, (including the Nucleus Accumbens), motor areas and networks involved in autonomic responses.

Thus, it would appear to be involved in the integration of emotion, cognition and behaviour.

ACC

As well as the Amygdala, the ACC has strong connections the Hippocampus and the Insula. The Insula (interoceptive information), the Hippocampus (context information), and the ACC form the 'saliency network' in determining what information gets preferential attention i.e. what information is most significant.

The ACC is significant in emotional regulation and in attention and has been shown to be one of the main areas influenced by mindfulness training.

Functional connections between the ACC and the Striatum are found to be impaired in Autistic Spectrum Disorders.

Spindle Cells in ACC

Spindle Cells, also known as Von Econommen Cells, or VEN cells, are found in the ACC, the Anterior Insula, and the Hippocampus. They are only found in animals with higher developed brains and are thought to underpin many functions of social behaviours.

These spindle cells develop post-natally and are not fully developed until adulthood. They are involved in:

- Spontaneity of behaviour.
- Emotional self-control and maturation including social insights.
- Self-control – this signal is almost absent in ADHD.
- Empathy towards others.
- May influence adult competence, or dysfunction, in emotional self-control.
- Problem solving.

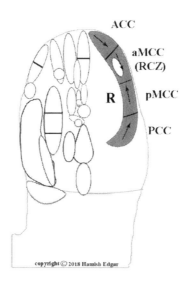

Cingulate Reflex Areas

Corpus Callosum

The Corpus Callosum is the broad band of fibres (White Matter) which exchange signals between the two hemispheres of the brain. It runs from the front to the back of the brain.

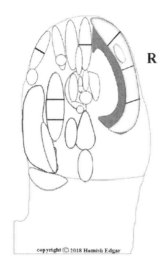

R

copyright © 2018 Hamish Edgar

Corpus Callosum Reflex Area

We would work this reflex area for Multiple Sclerosis and any condition where there is reduced white matter connections in the brain networks.

Midline Thalamus

The midline Thalamus nuclei play an important 'alerting' role in the detection of salient information. The midline Thalamus drives changes in attention and behaviour changes in response to changing external cues.

Anticipation of any gain/loss involves an 'alerting' signal from the Thalamus that combined with interoceptive information from the Insula, influences action selection in the NAc.

Reuniens (RE)

The RE nucleus is a midline Thalamus nucleus and is the major source of thalamic input to the Hippocampus.

Investigations into connections between the medial prefrontal cortex and the Hippocampus suggest that the Reuniens may be the principal route for the transfer of information from the mPFC to the Hippocampus.

The Reuniens may play an important role in the initiation of epileptic seizures and temporal lobe epilepsy.

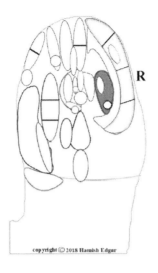

Midline Thalamus & Reuniens Reflex Areas

Habenula & Pineal

The Pineal and Habenula are collectively known as the Epithalamus.

Habenula

The Habenula is situated between the two Thalami towards the posterior above the pineal gland.

- The Habenula is involved in behavioural responses to pain, stress, anxiety, sleep and reward.
- The Habenula is hyperactive in depression, contributing to the generation of symptoms such as loss of motivation and anhedonia.
- Connected with the VTA/Substantia Nigra, Locus Coeruleus and Raphe Nucleus, and influences neurotransmitter release in those three areas.
- The Habenula is activated following non-delivery of expected reward and to aversive stimuli.
- Relay in descending pain modulation.
- Associated with tobacco, alcohol and cocaine addiction and withdrawal.

Pineal Gland

The level of light hitting the retina is detected by the SCN in the Hypothalamus. This triggers a cascade of signalling resulting in changes in the level of NE at the Pineal Gland. This in turn signals the enzymes involved in the two-stage process of conversion of Serotonin to Melatonin.

Melatonin is involved in many processes in the body.

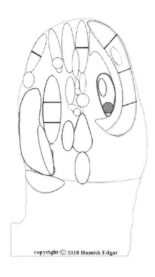

Epithalamus (Habenula & Pineal) Reflex Area

Cerebellum

The Cerebellum consists of two hemispheres and a narrow midline zone called the Vermis. Although the cerebellum represents only 10% volume of the brain, 60 to 80 % of the brain's neurons are found within the cerebellum.

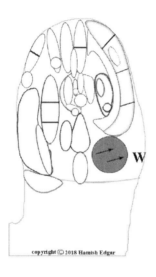

Cerebellum Reflex Area

Stress - a challenge to homeostasis.

External and internal sensory information reaches the brain through signalling pathways.

Through complex processes, the brain networks respond to this information in a way that is designed to maintain homeostatic norms.

Most of the time these processes are successful in restoring or maintaining homeostatic norms. However, in many conditions, problems arise when there are dysfunctional components within the networks affecting the homeostatic processes. For example, if there is loss of axon fibres, and thus reduced connectivity between areas of the brain networks, signals may not get through.

Many of these connections perform the regulatory functions of homeostasis. Where these regulatory networks are compromised by this deficient connectivity, this regulation is ineffective giving rise to imbalances in homeostatic norms.

Any deviation away from the body's homeostatic norms creates physiological stress.

Stress can be any form of threat to the body's integrity: situational, emotional, or physical such as an infection or illness. Anything that disturbs homeostasis beyond the acceptable limits will trigger a stress response.

When we say we are stressed we usually are referring to emotional stress or anxiety. This be a perceived inability to meet expectations whether these are expectations of others or expectations of ourselves.

Physical responses to emotional stress include:

- Sweating.
- Shaking.
- Immune response.
- Sense of exhaustion.

Cognitive (thinking) responses to emotional stress include:

- Perception that we have not got the resources to cope.
- Inability to focus attention.
- A wish to escape.
- Lowered mood or Depression.

We all know what stress feels like and what it looks like, but what creates the emotions that create the feeling of stress?

In the next section, we will explore the physiological processes that are at play and the role of the limbic brain.

The Stress Response

HPA Axis

One of the major responses to stress is the activation of the Hypothalamus-Pituitary-Adrenal Axis.

We have already discussed the Hypothalamus. We will take a brief look at the Pituitary and the Adrenal Glands.

Pituitary

The Pituitary is functionally connected to the Hypothalamus via a small tube called the infundibulum stem, or stalk.

The Anterior Pituitary receives its signals from the Hypothalamus in the form of releasing and inhibiting hormones. The effect of these hormones is to signal the Pituitary to start or stop producing the Anterior Pituitary hormones. The Posterior Pituitary receives its hormones directly via neuroendocrine neurons from the Hypothalamus.

Corticotrophin Releasing Hormone (CRH) is secreted by the Paraventricular nuclei in the Hypothalamus. This stimulates the synthesis of Adrenocorticotrophic Hormone (ACTH) in the Pituitary.

One of the targets of ACTH is the outer and middle layers of the Adrenal Cortex, where it induces the production of Aldosterone and Cortisol respectively, both important in the stress response.

Adrenal Glands (Suprarenal Glands)

The Adrenal Cortex

The Adrenal Cortex is composed of three layers, each secreting a distinct class of hormones; mineralocorticoids, glucocorticoids, and sex hormones.

The outer layer synthesises mineralocorticoids – mainly Aldosterone. Aldosterone influences the retention of salts in the kidney which in turn influences blood pressure.

The middle layer secretes glucocorticoids, steroids, mainly Cortisol.

The inner layer produces small quantities of the sex hormones oestrogen and testosterone - in both males and females.

Effects of Cortisol

- Increased availability of resources in response to stress.
- Breakdown of proteins.
- Increased production of glucose.
- Lipolysis (breakdown of fats for energy).
- Anti-inflammatory effect.
- Suppression, and redirection of the immune system (saving resources but also slowing healing).

Diurnal Cycle of Cortisol

The secretion of Cortisol follows a daily cycle with periods of increased and decreased secretion. It is highest on wakening reducing to its lowest level in the middle of the night.

In some conditions this cycle is disrupted. Some research indicates that in PTSD, the highs and lows are flattened out.

Adrenal Medulla

Whilst the Adrenal Cortex in under the control of the endocrine system, the Adrenal Medulla is part of the autonomic nervous system.

The Adrenal Medulla is also involved in the stress response through its involvement in the fight/flight response, where Chromaffin cells in the Adrenal Medulla are stimulated by the sympathetic division of the autonomic nervous system to secrete Epinephrine and Norepinephrine.

Effects of Epinephrine, and Norepinephrine

- Increase in heart rate and contraction.
- Increase in blood pressure.
- Increased blood flow to essential organs, skeletal muscle, and adipose tissue.
- Dilation of airways in lungs.
- Increased supply of glucose and fatty acids.

HPA feedback loop control

Under normal conditions the Hypothalamus monitors many chemicals in the circulating blood, including the circulating level of Cortisol. Depending on the level of Cortisol, the Hypothalamus responds by either increasing or reducing the secretion of CRH.

Control of HPA axis.

The axis is under excitable control by the Amygdala and Locus Coeruleus, and under inhibitory control by its inherent feedback loop and is regulated in part by the Hippocampus, Subiculum and BNST.

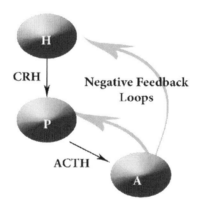

HPA Axis

Circuit chart of HPA

Stress and Anxiety treatments should also include all the relaxation reflex areas, e.g. Diaphragm and the spinal reflex area T9, which relates to the Adrenals.

Early life stress affects Hypothalamic Nuclei – for example, a set point or threshold is created in the Paraventricular Nucleus of the Hypothalamus for responding to Cortisol levels. Early traumatic experience will recalibrate this set point.

To determine the set point level of the number and sensitivity of glucocorticoid receptors in preparation for life outside the womb, the foetus takes its cue from the level of circulating Cortisol in the mother. This initial set point level will influence later responses to stress such as the responsiveness of the HPA Axis.

The HPA axis is the central processing motor that creates the physiological effects of stress, any physiological stress, not just emotional stress. It is a loop that not only generates the symptoms and signs of stress but is also involved in many other disease processes.

As any disturbance in homeostatic balance triggers the HPA, the HPA reflex areas should be worked in every treatment whatever the presenting problem.

Brain Gut Axis

Associated with the HPA axis is the Brain-Gut axis, which some cite as an explanation for IBS where chronic sub-clinical inflammation or infection in the bowel wall, triggers the HPA axis.

Eustress and Distress

Eustress refers to stress that triggers an adaptive response to circumstances.

Distress is maladaptive.

General Adaptation Syndrome

The General Adaptation Syndrome model is an attempt to describe and explain the nature of stress. The GAS describes three stages of the stress response.

General Adaptation Syndrome Stages:

Alarm.

The fight or flight response is an immediate survival response. The Hypothalamus stimulates the autonomic nervous system and the Adrenal Medulla.

Epinephrine has the effect of increasing blood supply to essential organs and skeletal muscle and reduces the blood supply to nonessential processes like digestion.

Resistance.

The resistance stage involves increased hormonal secretion of CRH, Gonadotrophin Hormone Releasing Hormone (GHRH) and Thyroid Releasing Hormone (TRH) - all releasing hormones from the Hypothalamus.

CRH, via the Pituitary and ACTH, stimulates production of Cortisol and Aldosterone in the Adrenal Cortex. GHRH and TRH prepare the body's resistance by their effects on blood pressure and electrolyte balance. Thus, hormonal processes prepare all the resources needed to deal with the continued stressor.

Exhaustion.

If these measures fail to deal with the stressor, resources become depleted resulting in pathological damage. Continued elevated levels of Cortisol secretion, amongst other things, limits the immune response and can lead to adrenal exhaustion and prolonged elevated blood pressure and can damage the function of the Hippocampus.

Acute Stress

Transient secretion of Cortisol and Epinephrine and Norepinephrine from the Adrenal Medulla.

Chronic Stress

With exposure to early life trauma or severe stress continuous stimulation of the HPA axis can become permanently hyperactive. This may establish higher basal ACTH and higher ACTH response to stress in adult life.

Chronic effects of Cortisol

- Changes to the immune system, leaving the individual vulnerable to infection.
- With chronic secretion there may be damage to the Hippocampus with loss of dendrites.
- Adrenal exhaustion.
- Down-regulation of Cortisol receptors (less sensitive).

In up-regulation the receptors become hypersensitive, so a low level of Cortisol will trigger a response.

In down-regulation the numbers of receptors are reduced, so the Hypothalamus becomes hyposensitive.

Emotions and how they arise.

Emotions are the physical manifestations of the response of the brain to information. Feelings are the conscious perceptions, or awareness, of those emotions.

The prime purpose of emotions is to attach personal significance to information and to mobilise appropriate physiological, and behavioural, responses that best ensures our survival. As we shall see, there are networks that prioritise information – information, whose significance demands precedence for attention.

Any conscious perception of information has a personal meaning and significance. A person's memories and prior experience can colour the interpretation of the incoming stimuli. And so, the context of the information will influence an individual's emotional response.

How then do we know what emotion we are feeling?

What is the difference between love and anger? How do we decide what to call the feeling? What are the physical cues?

MRI images tell us, that different emotions affect different parts of the brain and that those areas do not overlap.

Embodied Cognition.

In the nineteenth century, William James, a pre-eminent American Psychologist, offered the theory of 'Embodied Cognition' to answer these questions.

Conventionally, we think that the physical sensations of emotion arise from our thoughts and our appraisal of any given situation. We think something is sad, therefore we cry.

James believed that this was not necessarily a one-way process. He suggested that the physical sensations of emotion might come first. Only then do we attach a meaning to the sensations. So, signals from the autonomic nervous system may shape our emotional experience.

According to the theory of embodied cognition, we become afraid because we are shaking, and our stomach is churning.

Memory & Learning

Clients rarely seek help for pleasurable memories, so we are particularly interested in the neural networks of emotional fear. Here we will explore the neurobiology of memory and fear memory.

To understand memory, we need to understand the process that we call learning.

Earlier we learned about synapses and neurotransmitters. As we explore fear memory, we will discover that changes in synapses underpin the neurobiology of learning and memory.

So, what exactly in neurological terms is a memory?

To answer this question, we need to learn about conditioning, synaptic plasticity and the four processes involved in memory.

Classical Conditioning

In Classical Conditioning, a neutral innocuous event is paired with an aversive event such as pain. We learn to associate one with the other so that the innocuous event on its own, elicits an emotional or behavioural response.

This type of learning is sometimes referred to as Pavlonian learning. Pavlov's dog learned to salivate to the sound of a bell. When presented with food, the dog salivated. Pavlov sounded a bell at the same time as presenting the food and the sound of the bell came to be associated with food, so that over time the dog would salivate when the bell was sounded, even in the absence of food.

Convergence of conditioned stimulus (CS), and unconditioned stimuli (US) occur in the Amygdala. Both the CS and the US converge on the same synapse in the Amygdala, thus they become associated.

Extinction of the response occurs when the innocuous event happens for several occasions without the aversive event, and so the association with the aversive event is diminished.

Operant Conditioning

In Operant Conditioning we learn to associate an action or behaviour with a reward. We learn this by trial and error.

All our behaviours have consequential outcomes. We learn that the outcome follows the behaviour. Every time I press the button the lift opens.

Operant conditioning depends on a reward for the behaviour.

This is sometimes referred to as instrumental learning – you learn to use specific behaviours as an instrument to gain a reward or a desired outcome.

We also learn to behave in such a way as to avoid an aversive consequence or a negative reward.

Arousal strengthens memory.

All learning is enhanced depending on the state of arousal at the time of learning. If we are not emotionally aroused during the experience, then learning is diminished.

Therefore, we can vividly remember emotionally charged events easier, such as fearful memories. We learn them better because of the heightened emotional arousal at the time.

As we shall discover, this is down to a sequence of reactions involving stress hormones, the Locus Coeruleus, and the Amygdala.

Synaptic plasticity and Learning

We have established that chemical and electrical signals are involved in the communication between neighbouring neurons, and that this occurs at synapses.

We learned that signals cross the synaptic cleft and bind with receivers - the receptors - on the neighbouring neuron.

We also learned that this activity at the synapse could either be excitatory or inhibitory.

Synaptic plasticity is the ability of synapses to undergo lasting modifications after repeated stimulation and experience. (Plastic in this sense, simply means changeable).

These lasting modifications include:

- An increase in the strength of the signals.
- An increase in the numbers of receptors on the post-synaptic neuron.

Synaptic plasticity underpins the neurological process involved in learning, memory, and habitual thought.

The plastic changes that increase strength of the signal and the number of receptors in learning is referred to as Long Term Potentiation (LTP). The signal lasts longer and the receptors are more numerous.

Plastic changes, like those mentioned above, occur at the synapses when a neuron is repeatedly fired. When the same set of neurons fire repeatedly together, they get used to firing together in sequence. They have 'learned'. This is the basis of memory.

So, what we call memory turns out to be well-trodden neural pathways.

The converse is, that over a period, if these synapses are not used, then the strength of the signal falls and there is a reduction in the number of post-synaptic receptors.

When this happens, it is referred to as Long Term Depression (LTD).

It's a case of use it or lose it. If not used, the 'memory' fades.

Types of Memory

Memory can be subdivided into, Short Term Memory and Long-Term Memory

Short Term Memory, or Working Memory, is transient - shopping list, where we put our keys, etc.

Long-Term Memory can be subdivided into Implicit, and Explicit Memory.

Implicit Memory

All our habits engage Implicit Memory. We learn manual skills through Implicit Memory. Riding a bike, tying shoelaces, driving the same route to work.

Implicit Memory is sometimes referred to as declarative, or procedural memory.

Explicit or Episodic Memory

These are memories of events and facts - the conscious recall of information about people, places and objects. Explicit memory is involved when we store facts and episodes, hence episodic or autobiographical memory.

Four processes involved in memory

1. Encoding.
2. Storage.
3. Consolidation.
4. Retrieval.

Encoding

New information is mainly processed in the Hippocampus. This new information gets linked to what we already know by comparing and classifying new information.

Storage

It is unclear where memories reside. Memories have various components including sights, sounds, and smells, so the storage of memories is widespread throughout the brain - in the visual, auditory and olfactory brain areas. Cues tap into these associations. A word can has many associations. e.g. the word elephant can have associations with - grey, living things, memory of the zoo, size, trumpeting sound, circus, savannah etc. and all the visual, auditory, olfactory and emotional associations that each of us have.

As we know, emotionally charged episodic memories, including fear memories, involve specific activation of the Amygdala.

Consolidation

This involves strengthening of synapses with repeated stimulation. This process converts short term memory into longer term memory. We tend to consolidate significant information. We tend not to consolidate insignificant information such as last week's shopping list.

Retrieval

When retrieved, a memory becomes sensitive to change - becomes more plastic - and when plastic, relearning can take place.

Deliberately not retrieving memories is therefore an ineffective way of dealing with painful memory. It does not allow these memories to become plastic and thus precludes relearning.

'Sins' of memory

Memories are notoriously unreliable. That is because over time, they can become distorted.

Blocking - 'tip of tongue' phenomenon

Misattribution - associating memory with wrong details such as time or place i.e. false memory. In the Hippocampus, false memories utilise the same pathways as accurate memories. This is why false memories seem so real.

Suggestibility - memories can become biased or distorted to fit with our current beliefs – we distort memory to avoid conflict with our beliefs.

Persistence - memories may become intrusive in our thoughts. The memory pops into our head without being invited. This is a common feature of OCD and PTSD.

Limbic areas involvement in learning and memory

Memory circuits are very complex. There are many networks and nuclei involved in what we call memory. We are interested in the involvement of those nuclei for which we have corresponding reflex areas.

Hippocampus

The Hippocampus is pivotal in new learning. It is involved in all the stages of learning. Any deficits in the Hippocampus will impact on the efficiency of memory and learning.

Amygdala

As we saw, the Amygdala stores episodic fear memories. These are thought to reside in the Basolateral area (BLA) of the Amygdala which when activated, in turn activates the Central Amygdala Nucleus (CE) which is the main output area from the Amygdala.

In Classical Conditioning there is convergence of the conditioned (tone), and unconditioned stimuli (pain), on the same neurons in the BLA, leading to synaptic plasticity, thus the tone and the pain become associated.

The Central Amygdala (CE) connects with the Hypothalamus (hormonal responses) and brainstem areas like the PAG that control the expression of conditioned fear response. This would include freezing. (autonomic nervous system)

(Morphine administration impairs the consolidation of the memory through its effects on the Amygdala. Those receiving morphine immediately after a life-threatening event are less likely to develop PTSD)

Locus Coeruleus

Involved in arousal circuits and sleep-awake cycles. Learning is enhanced with elevated arousal and influences the consolidation of long-term memory. Stress hormones like Epinephrine and Cortisol influence the Locus Coeruleus via the Vagus Nerve.

Increases in the release of Norepinephrine from the Locus Coeruleus augments memory processing at synapses throughout the brain. Thus, in arousal states, the experience is remembered better.

Norepinephrine is also involved in plastic changes in the Hippocampus in dampening down older memories (LTD) when new information needs to take precedence.

Memory extinction – Forgetting, or learning again

One of the major problems in PTSD is the failure to extinguish fear memory or failure to downgrade the emotional response to those memories.

Memory formation is associated with initial encoding to establish a short-term memory (STM) followed by a time-dependent consolidation phase to establish a stable long-term memory (LTM).

Retrieval of LTM destabilizes, or deconsolidates the memory, rendering it labile once more. For the LTM to become re-established, it requires reconsolidation following retrieval.

Failure to reconsolidate the memory trace results in decay of that memory, much as STM decays in the absence of consolidation (last week's shopping list).

So, remembering or retrieving a memory creates the opportunity to change the memory, or create an alternative take on the event.

So, extinction does not actually erase the original troublesome memory. Rather, retrieval allows new learning about the event.

Thus, in fear memory, new learning can create a new memory that competes with and inhibits the fear memory, which can lead to altered behavioural responses to the memory of the event.

Most therapies employed in the treatment of PTSD are designed to reconstruct memories in this fashion. EMDR, and exposure therapies involve the use of mental imagery and exposure to trauma-relevant cues in a safe environment to suppress the fear associated with the memory of the traumatic event.

Fear conditioning and fear extinction are encoded in the Amygdala, and contextual retrieval cues determine which memory is expressed in behaviour.

The Medial Prefrontal Cortex and Hippocampus are involved in processing contextual information, (where it happened and what else was going on at the time), and both have rich connections with the Amygdala, suggesting that the PFC and Hippocampus play a role in establishing extinction memories.

Pain

Introduction

As a large proportion of our clients present with pain conditions, we will look at pain in detail.

As we explore the basic physiology of pain and how pain is processed and perceived, we will discover that there is significant overlap between the pathways and processes of pain and the networks involved in emotion.

Because of this shared underlying physiology, we will discover that emotional processing has a significant impact on our perception of pain and vice versa.

Pain may be defined as an unpleasant sensory or emotional experience, with actual or potential tissue damage.

It has urgency about it and so gets preferential attention. Pain is also subjective, and the perception of pain can vary across time in any one individual and is influenced by many factors and complex neural processes.

We need to feel pain. Pain alerts us to injuries that require either evasion or treatment and so fulfils a protective function.

Whilst acute pain triggers an immediate response, persistent pain motivates us to get appropriate treatment. Chronic pain however, has no useful purpose.

Chronic pain is probably the single most common condition that Reflexologists are asked to treat. There are already effective mainstream treatments to address pain. Limbic Reflexology adds to those, by addressing the processes that underlie the chronicity of the condition.

Limbic Reflexology gives us access to central processes such as sensitisation - the plastic changes that underlie the processes that transform acute pain into chronic pain conditions.

Ascending pathways are involved in the perception of pain and the descending pathways are involved in the facilitation of pain and the inhibitory controls that the brain exerts on the transmission of pain signals.

The Physiology of Pain

Nociception

Pain is perceived in the brain. Pain signals are transmitted from the site of injury to the Central Nervous System through neural pathways. This is called nociception.

Peripheral processes and Central processes

Peripheral, refers to the pathway from the tissues to the spinal cord.

Central, refers to the pathway from the spinal cord to the brain.

The Peripheral Process of Pain

The peripheral process involves nociceptors and receptor neurons.

Nociceptors are simply bare nerve endings.

There are four types of nociceptors.

- Thermal. Responsive to change in temperature.
- Mechanical. Responsive to touch and pressure.
- Polymodal. Responsive to a variety of stimuli.
- Silent – mainly in internal organs.

Nociceptors have two main types of fibres or axons.

A-delta fibres

These are thinly myelinated and have a low threshold (easily stimulated). Because they are myelinated, they transmit signals faster.

C - fibres

These are unmyelinated, with a high threshold. Signal transmission in these fibres is slower as they are unmyelinated.

When we stub our toe, there is a first sharp pain, followed a few moments by an aching throbbing pain.

The first sharp pain – thermal and mechanical signals, are conveyed by A-delta fibres – fast pain.

The second, aching burning pain, is conveyed by C fibres – slower pain.

There are a range of receptors involved in nociception and each receptor has a different threshold. This is the point at which it is activated.

For example, in temperature perception, each thermal receptor is activated by varying degrees of temperature.

Low threshold receptors require less stimulation to activate them, high threshold receptors need more stimulation to become activated.

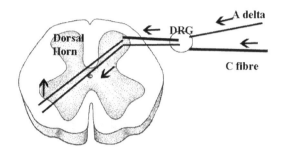

Section of the Spinal Cord

The A delta fibres and C fibres project onto the dorsal root ganglion (DRG), and on to various locations of the dorsal horn of the spinal cord. The signals are now in the CNS.

From here, the signals cross over to the other side to the anterior white fibres of the cord, and the signals get transmitted up various tracts, or pathways to the brain where they are eventually perceived in the brain as pain.

Immune System & Pain

At the site of the injury and at the level of the spinal cord, there are many other biochemical influences on nociception.

At any site of injury to tissue, there collects a 'soup' of chemicals. These include proteins and cytokines, amassed by the immune system in response to injury, which triggers inflammation.

Nociceptors, like all receptors, have a point where they respond. This is referred to as their threshold.

Cytokines, have the effect of lowering this threshold, making them more sensitive and increasing the pain response.

Oedema and inflammation triggers pain.

Inflammation stimulates the release of neuropeptides such as Substance P (SP). Substance P, as well as causing local vasodilation, lowers the threshold of nociceptors further which leads to the increased activation of A delta and C fibres.

SP also activates degranulation of mast cells which further excites nociceptors by reducing their threshold.

As we shall see, in Fibromyalgia Substance P is often found to be abnormally elevated.

Central Processes of Pain

From the spinal cord, signals travel up to the brain via various white fibre pathways.

The pathway for nociception is called the Spinothalamic Tract, which as its name suggests conveys pain signals from the spine to the Thalamus. These signals are then relayed to other areas of the brain, including limbic areas.

Two parallel pathways of the Spinothalamic tract – Lateral and Medial

The Lateral spinothalamic tract constitutes the sensory dimension of pain. This tract projects to the Thalamus, and then to the sensory cortex.

The Medial spinothalamic tract projects via the brainstem and medial Thalamus, then goes to the limbic regions thus eliciting the emotional and autonomic responses to pain.

Although it seems counterintuitive, we can see that pain is not perceived at the site of injury but in the brain. When the nociceptive pathways are blocked, e.g. by anaesthetics, then we cannot 'feel' the injury.

Pain Inhibition

The body has several processes that it employs in its response to pain, both at the level of the spinal cord and in the higher levels of the CNS.

Peripheral Convergence and Gate Control Inhibition

Projection neurons at the dorsal horn are activated by afferent (incoming) neurons which results in a convergence of signals at the spinal cord.

Some dorsal root ganglia receive convergent inputs from both nociceptive and non-nociceptive neurons. This sets up a competition between signals.

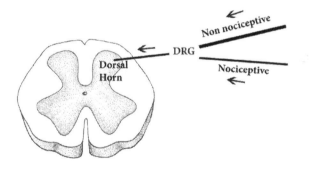

Nociceptive neurons are of a small diameter, whilst other non-nociceptive neurons have large diameters. In the competition for predominance, large fibre non-pain neurons can block the pain signals from the smaller diameter fibres.

Rubbing the site of an injury activates large mechanical fibres. This closes the gate to nociception, leading to lowered transmission and perception of pain. This is also the rationale underlying the TENS machine.

Central inhibition

In the CNS, pain is inhibited firstly by descending inhibitory pathways, and secondly by descending analgesia pathways and endogenous opiates. (endogenous = from within)

Inhibitory pathways

One inhibitory pathway has origins in the Anterior Cingulate Cortex, Hypothalamus and Amygdala.

This pathway stimulates nuclei in the Periaqueductal Grey which project signals to the Raphe Magnus in the Medulla.

The Raphe Magnus Nuclei in turn, project signals to the dorsal horn of the spinal cord, stimulating the release of Serotonin.

The Raphe is the main source of Serotonin in the CNS. This Serotonin inhibits the transmission of nociceptive signals, by suppressing the production of substance P in the spinal cord.

Descending Serotonin neurons have a widespread distribution in the spinal cord, so in chronic pain, diminished Serotonin is likely to result in widespread pain.

Independently, there are projections from the Locus Coeruleus directly to the dorsal horn in the spinal cord. As we know, projections from the Locus Coeruleus release Noradrenaline.

The LC can have either an Inhibitory or a facilitatory influence on the transmission of pain signals from the spinal cord.

There are two types of Noradrenaline receptors in the dorsal horn - alpha1 receptors and alpha2 receptors.

Signals to alpha1 receptors are facilitatory, that is they facilitate nociception. Signals to dorsal horn alpha2 receptors are inhibitory, that is, when activated, pain signals are inhibited.

So, in peripheral inhibition, Serotonin inhibits the transmission of nociceptive signals by suppressing the production of Substance P, and Norepinephrine activates alpha2 receptors at the dorsal horn which inhibits pain signals.

Inhibitory Pathways

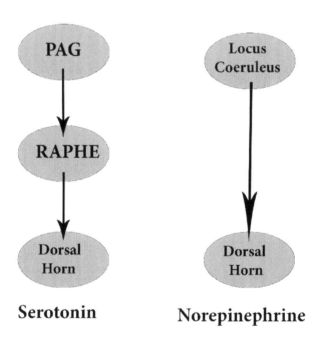

Descending Analgesia, and Endogenous Opiates (endogenous = from within)

In response to nociception, the body releases natural opiates. Beta-endorphins are one of the main endogenous opiates and some are synthesised in the Pituitary and released into the blood.

Some neurons in the Hypothalamus and macrophages in the immune system also synthesise endorphins and Beta-endorphins.

The Amygdala and ACC are very much involved in endogenous opioid analgesia, so in conditions where there is loss of descending analgesia, the Amygdala and ACC are important reflex areas to work.

Opioid Receptors

Opiates bind to presynaptic receptors, inhibiting the release of neurotransmitters, thus blocking nociceptive signals and reducing the activity of the postsynaptic neuron.

There are four classes of opiate receptors, the most diverse being μ (mu) receptors which are widespread and are heavily concentrated in the PAG and the dorsal horn of the spinal column. These receptors bind with opiates and endorphins.

When stimulated by endogenous opiates such as beta-endorphin, opioid receptors in the spinal cord and PAG inhibit pain by Influencing signal transmission from the dorsal horn to the CNS. Norepinephrine from the Locus Coeruleus enhances this effect of opioids.

Cannabinoids

Cannabinoids are not opiates but are another class of analgesics. They reduce both glutamate and GABA release.

Their action is a retrograde process at synapses and go in the opposite direction to neurotransmitters. That is, whereas neurotransmitters are released by the presynaptic neurons and cross to the postsynaptic neuron, cannabinoids are released by the postsynaptic neuron and cross to the presynaptic neuron.

They inhibit the action of presynaptic vesicles thus preventing the release of presynaptic neurotransmitters.

The Rostral Ventromedial Medulla (RVM) is an area running the length of the Medulla. There are complex processes within the RVM which influences nociception. In the RVM there are 'on cells' which promote pain signals, and 'off cells' that block or inhibit pain signals.

If activated 'on cells' predominate, this will result in a facilitatory effect with an increase in pain. If activated 'off cells' predominate, then there is an inhibitory effect and reduced pain. It is thought that in chronic pain, this process gets stuck in the facilitatory mode.

Cannabis is a Cannabinoid derived from plant material.

Cannabinoids, and endogenous opioids bind with opiate receptors in the RVM. They inhibit the 'on' cells and disinhibit the 'off' cells, thus reducing the transmission of pain signals.

Emotion and perception of pain

Now we know the physiological processes involved in pain perception and pain control, we will look at processes that control our emotional responses and the limbic networks that are involved in the emotional response to pain. Both emotional and cognitive responses influence the experience of pain.

Attention to pain

Because of its salience, its significance for survival, pain automatically gets preferential information processing at the expense of other information.

The Anterior Cingulate Cortex(ACC), Insula, and Locus Coeruleus(LC) are heavily involved in determining attention. Pain experience varies according to this attention– when attention is focused on pain, pain becomes more intense. Conversely, when focus of attention is distracted, the pain is less intense. This is the concept that underlies meditation and mindfulness (Discussed later).

In chronic pain conditions, attention to pain can become hypervigilant. Hypervigilance to harmful pain can lead to moderate painful stimuli being interpreted as more painful.

So, working the Saliency network reflex areas should impact on the attentional aspect of pain

Cognitive appraisal

Habitual emotional reactions, which are called cognitive styles, influence our experience of pain. These include catastrophizing and hypervigilance

Emotional reaction affects intensity

As we know, with negative emotion there is increased activity in the Amygdala, Insula, Prefrontal Cortex and Anterior Cingulate Cortex. These are also involved in the pain networks or matrix.

Heightened emotional activity therefore amplifies attention to pain, amplifies body awareness and pain unpleasantness, and lowers the expectation of the ability to cope with pain.

We have already seen that increased attention and a perception of poor control over pain, increases the intensity of pain.

Pain and Fear

Fear is a response to present threat - anxiety is the anticipation of real or imagined threat.

Fear inhibits pain due to activation of endogenous opioids. An evolutionary explanation for this is that it gains temporary postponement of disabling pain until it is safe to do so. Anxiety increases pain leading to a hypervigilance for pain. Repeated fear can lead to anxiety and increased sensitivity to pain.

Conversely, positive emotional states reduce pain.

Pain for gain.

The perception of pain is reduced when there is a conflicting motivation - pain for gain. Something more pressing or important makes it worthwhile tolerating the pain.

Unresolved stressors increase sensitivity to pain

In PTSD, persistent pain is common.

Emotional Expressiveness

There is a link between emotional expression / suppression with pain experience. People who tend to express their feelings experience lower pain, and those who are more aware of their emotional experience or reflect on their emotions have a higher tolerance of pain.

Behaviour responses to pain

In chronic pain, avoiding situations that make the pain worse can lead to avoidance as a coping strategy. This can lead to fear of pain and hypervigilance and a vicious cycle becomes established.

Avoidance, and beliefs about coping abilities, can lead to a lifestyle of functional disability, which is more associated with fear avoidance than pain severity.

With an apparent absence of any obvious disease, this can lead to the label of malingering or somatisation, a common label formally attached to unexplained conditions such as Fibromyalgia or M.E. ('yuppie flu').

Pain and the Limbic Brain

Insula

The Insula is highly activated in pain. We know that the posterior Insula receives sensory information from the Thalamus. Through this, the Insula acquires an awareness of the internal bodily states and thus is said to have interoceptive awareness. The Posterior Insula measures the intensity of pain. (The dorsal Cingulate measures the unpleasantness of pain)

The Posterior Insula projects to the Anterior Insula which is involved in initiating an appropriate emotional response. This is fed to the ACC, where an appropriate autonomic and behaviour response is initiated.

Amygdala

The Amygdala is activated by threat which includes pain. It receives direct projections from the brainstem and is involved in the activation of the HPA and in the reward/aversion circuits. It is also strongly involved in descending analgesia.

Hippocampus

The Hippocampus is involved in memory and especially the context component of memory. The Hippocampus is central to learning and long-term potentiation (LTP). This involves extensive plastic changes and in forming new neurons - neurogenesis. In chronic pain, there are plastic changes in the Hippocampus.

Subiculum

There are direct projections from the Subiculum to the prefrontal areas of the cortex. These projections induce long-term plasticity of nociceptive responses of PFC neurons. The Subiculum also helps regulate the HPA axis.

HPA Axis

The HPA is activated by stress and threat and initiates autonomic and endocrine responses to threat, including pain and the emotional responses to pain.

Pituitary

In addition to its endocrine role in the HPA axis, the Pituitary produces endogenous opiates such as endorphins which are involved in the inhibition of pain.

Adrenals

Cortisol, produced by the Adrenals, is involved in the inhibition of the inflammatory response to injury. Cortisol receptors are widespread in the brain, and Cortisol plays a major role in regulating responses.

Striatum & Nucleus Accumbens

As we know, the Nucleus Accumbens is involved in reward circuits and has two modes; approach and aversion.

Pain will trigger the aversion mode whereas analgesia represents reward (reduced pain). The Nucleus Accumbens is highly activated in anticipation of pain (and relief of pain). In placebo research involving anticipated analgesia (reward), the Nucleus Accumbens is highly activated.

Anterior Cingulate Cortex

The ACC has a pivotal role in influencing our perception and response to pain. As we learned above, along with the Anterior Insula, the ACC forms the core of the Saliency Network.

As such, it has a role in determining the significance of events thus the information that demands our attention. It is thought to be involved both in the attention to pain and in the preparation and initiation of appropriate autonomic and behavioural responses to pain.

The ACC has reciprocal connections with the Nucleus Accumbens and rich connections with the motor cortex, the Amygdala, the Thalamus and the PAG. The autonomic response will include such things as heart rate and the behavioural responses will involve aversive behaviours (Nucleus Accumbens in aversive mode), and the initiation of movement (Striatum).

The Cingulate is not involved in the perception of the intensity of pain (Insula), but in the level of unpleasantness, or the suffering aspect of pain. It has been demonstrated that the ACC is the main area influenced by meditation and mindfulness, which influences attention to pain and thus the unpleasantness rating of pain.

The ACC is also involved in the acquisition of fear memory. This includes memory of pain.

Prefrontal Cortex

The PFC is central to processing cognitive responses to pain, and in evaluating the personal meaning of body sensations – 'Have I the resources to cope with it?'

Pain intensity is reduced when it is perceived to be controllable.

Pain intensity is increased where it is seen as potentially overwhelming – not controllable. The PFC regulates this perception.

The emotional dimension of pain involves fear memories formed by pain experiences. The PFC is involved in forming the emotional memory of pain. Plastic changes in the PFC may also underlie the phenomena of phantom pain. The pain is remembered.

Locus Coeruleus

As well as nociceptive information going to the Thalamus, the LC receives information directly from the dorsal horn of the spinal cord. Pain, like all stressors stimulates release of Norepinephrine from LC. As we have seen, Norepinephrine is heavily involved both in direct inhibition of pain and in a supporting role in descending analgesia.

In the management of chronic pain, many analgesic drugs exert their effect by raising the levels of Norepinephrine, e.g. Amitriptyline.

Chronic Pain

Chronic Pain results from one or more of the following:

- Impaired descending analgesia.
- Impaired inhibitory pathways.
- Enhanced facilitation pathway.
- Peripheral and/or Central Sensitisation.

Hyperalgesia and Allodynia

Two features of chronic pain are Hyperalgesia and Allodynia.

Hyperalgesia is where a painful stimulus is perceived as more painful than it should be.

Allodynia is a perception of pain resulting from a stimulus that would not normally be painful.

Impaired descending analgesia

The Amygdala is strongly involved in opioid dependant analgesia by its activation of PAG processes.

In chronic pain, there are plastic changes in the Amygdala, which impairs its role in descending analgesia. There are also changes in the brainstem which alters the responsiveness of the opioid receptors, leading to a predominance of activated 'on cells'.

Impaired Inhibitory Pathway and / or enhanced Facilitation Pathway

Serotonin is reduced in chronic pain, which points to impairment of the Raphe function. Since Serotonin inhibits the pain signal transmission at the dorsal horn, depletion of available Serotonin will lead to the dorsal horn pathways becoming overexcited. If the Norepinephrine inhibitory pathway is impaired, the LC may get stuck in the facilitatory mode.

Gate Control Inhibition

At the spinal cord level, there may be a loss of gate control inhibition leading to hyperalgesia.

Wind up and Summation

Wind up and Summation is a mechanism in which repetitive noxious stimulation results in a slow build-up effect, or summation, that is experienced as increased pain. The perception of pain thus becomes disproportionate to the degree of injury.

Summation is thought to be a major contributory feature in Fibromyalgia and in chronic tension-type headache (CTH) patients.

Central Sensitisation

Repeated firing of C fibres and chronic activation of the peripheral pain receptors can lead to habituation (decreased response), or sensitization (increased response) of pain receptors.

These changes in receptors involve plastic changes like those involved in learning and memory, so that sensitisation could be a form of learning. Persistent stimulation creates a well-trodden neural path.

In chronic pain conditions, peripheral or central sensitisation leads to lower thresholds for excitation or to spontaneous pain e.g. phantom pain following amputation.

Sensitisation can occur in any region. In chronic or persistent pain there may be plastic changes to the Insula, Amygdala, Hippocampus, LC, ACC, OFC, Striatum, Hypothalamus, Thalamus and PAG.

Central sensitisation often results in cross sensitisation. This means that as pain and emotion share common circuits, nociceptor signals will impact on emotions and vice versa. Chronic pain is often accompanied by Depression and Anxiety and Depression impacts on the perception of pain.

Reflex Areas in chronic pain

So, we find that all of the limbic reflex areas have some relevance in chronic pain conditions:

In addition, where there is an inflammatory component, the Lymphatic Spine and Thymus may be worked.

The focus of the treatment will of course be guided by the presenting condition and by the maxim,' work what you find to be tender.'

See Appendix A for Medication, commonly prescribed for chronic pain conditions.

Mindfulness and Meditation

Attention to the moment (mindfulness), involves activity in the Prefrontal Cortex, Cingulate Cortex, the Insula and the Locus Coeruleus.

The Insula integrates external, internal, and body state information.

The ACC and aMCC coordinates appropriate responses and are heavily involved in attention.

The LC is the main source of Noradrenaline in the brain and is central to arousal and attention (Central Noradrenaline).

The LC also exerts influence on the Nucleus Ambiguous (NA) in the Medulla. The Nucleus Ambiguous consists of the Cranial Nerves IX & X, which control heart rate and other processes of the sympathetic nervous system. Thus, by manipulating both central and peripheral Noradrenaline, the LC can adapt the state of the whole organism to optimise attention.

We have already seen that when the focus of attention is distracted, pain is less intense. So, focussing on the moment (mindfulness) or focussing on an internal image or object has the effect of reducing the perception of pain.

Networks.

Saliency Network

The Saliency network mainly consists of the Insula, Hippocampus, and the Cingulate.

Between them, the significance of information is established. The significance is based on the perceived threat to homeostasis. The significance of stimuli will vary from one individual to another, depending on experience.

The Insula as we know, monitors both internal and external environments. The Hippocampus compares this information with the contextual memory of similar information and the Cingulate integrates this information into an appropriate action plan.

Salient or significant information will receive preferential attention at the expense of less salient information. Pain information for example, will automatically get preferential attention.

Default Mode Network and Central Executive Network

Two other networks that are commonly referred to are the Default Mode Network (DMN) and the Central Executive Network (CEN).

The Default Mode Network is more activated when we are not engaged with tasks and so is associated with internally generated thoughts, self-referential thinking, autobiographical memories and ruminating thoughts.

Amongst others, the ACC and PCC are parts of this network.

When we engage in task related activity and thinking, we switch to the Central Executive Network.

When we keep ourselves busy doing something to stop ourselves from thinking about a traumatic memory or issue, we are probably preventing the switch to DMN and activation of PCC.

It is thought that the Insula and pgACC are the main areas that are involved in switching from one Network to the other.

Failure to switch effectively may underpin problems of concentration and lack of engagement common in mood disorders and the "fog" of Fibromyalgia.

Common Conditions

Sleep

Many of our clients have problems with sleeping. We all know that insomnia disrupts our functioning. Often, insomnia comes as part of another condition, such as chronic pain or Depression.

The purpose of sleep is much debated, but what is known, is that it serves several functions. All animals sleep. Even sharks, who must be constantly on the move to breathe, sleep with one half of their brain at a time. Amongst other things, sleep helps memory consolidation and learning. Lack of sleep affects cognition (thinking), judgement, the perception of pain, and severely affects our mood.

What is known to a large extent, are the networks involved in sleep/wake states. Throughout the brainstem, there are networks that make up the Reticular Activating System (RAS). Put simply, the RAS 'wakens' the brain. Sleep/wake states involve complex processes involving many of the areas we are now familiar with, including the Raphe Nucleus, PAG, Thalamus, Locus Coeruleus, PFC, Hypothalamus and Hippocampus.

The initiation of sleep involves many of the Hypothalamic nuclei, most notably the SCN, LHA, Preoptic and the TMN.

Like all animals, our brain responds to light levels. Photosensitive cells in the retina send information directly to the Suprachiasmic Nucleus of the Hypothalamus. When light levels fall, the Suprachiasmic Nucleus, through the autonomic nervous system, triggers a cascade of processes that induces sleep.

One of those processes involves an increase in the supply of Norepinephrine to the Pineal gland, which stimulates an increase in the synthesis of Melatonin which is involved in the promotion of sleep in humans.

Bizarrely, in nocturnal animals, Melatonin is also increased in low light, but this has the opposite effect of stimulating wakefulness. Light levels also initiate breeding cycles and hibernation in animals.

The Suprachiasmic Nucleus is the master clock of circadian rhythms. All the 'clocks' of the body, and there many of them, set their time to the Suprachiasmic Nucleus. For example, in the endocrine system, hormones secrete in a circadian fashion. So, working the Hypothalamus, and specifically the SCN, is appropriate in problems involving reproduction as well as sleep problems.

Anxiety

Anxiety is seen as a long-term trait with hypervigilance, and where the potential for threat in uncertain and unpredictable situations is habitually overestimated.

Fear is seen as a heightened arousal towards an immediate and predictable threat.

The BNST is active during anxiety and unpredictable threat, but not in fear, which happens when faced with predictable threat.

The Amygdala is the opposite. It becomes active when faced with predictable threat but not when faced with unpredictable threat.

The BNST is composed of several sub-nuclei and they regulate anxiety in opposite directions. Some increase anxiety, whilst others decreases anxiety.

We know the sgACC helps regulate the Amygdala. In addition, the Subgenual Cingulate also influences the BNST.

The Amygdala and the BNST project to the Hypothalamus and to brain stem areas which modulate various features of anxiety such as heart rate and respiratory rate. Activity in the BNST also influences the stress response of the HPA.

So, the sgACC, the Hippocampus, the Amygdala and BNST, constitute a network which when coordinated controls and regulates anxiety.

Depression

We are all used to using the words mood and depression in our everyday description of how we feel. However, in the context of psychological well-being, these concepts assume a more precise meaning. Mood is often referred to as affect. Euthymic, refers to the 'normal' cycle of ups and downs, that we can all identify with. We may feel optimistic and positive one day, and on another day, we can be pessimistic, and disinterested in things that we normally would be enthusiastic about.

Cyclothymia however, describes swings in this cycle which may persist for weeks or months. The swings however, are not so severe as those found in Depression.

Depression as a disorder, describes a basketful of problems, of which lowering of mood is only one. It is a short hand way of describing the items in the basket. Each person's Depression may differ in the significance and range of items in the basket.

The problems may include lowered mood, anhedonia, or getting little or no pleasure in things that they used to enjoy, loss of interest, sleep and appetite disturbance, feelings of low self-worth, ruminating thoughts about self, focusing on negative events, difficulty in recognising positive events, an unjustified sense of guilt, sense of poverty and ideas of self-harm or not wanting to be here.

We can all experience some of these at one time or another without being depressed. What determines Depression is the presence of a collection of these features over a period of time. To satisfy the criteria of

Major Depressive Disorder, DSM states this duration to be a minimum of one month.

Statistics suggest that one in four of us are likely to experience Clinical Depression at least once in our lifetime, and three quarters of those will be prone to recurring episodes.

Depression is often found to occur alongside other conditions such as chronic pain or Anxiety, and when we look at the networks affected in each of them, we see that there are extensive shared networks in the conditions.

In Major Depression Disorder (MDD), functional abnormalities and structural differences have been identified in a wide range of areas. Functional changes contribute to diminished cognitive control and biased information processing with biased processing of emotional stimuli. There is heightened response to negative emotional stimuli and a corresponding reduction in response to positive stimuli, suggesting an attentional bias towards information that is seen as negative.

Evidence suggests that in MDD there is decreased oligodendrocytes and reduced white matter, resulting in dysfunctional connections in the limbic areas, including the PFC, Thalamus and Corpus Callosum. Early de-myelination is associated with the severity of MDD.

Deficits in working memory compromise the ability to carry out routine tasks efficiently.

The PFC, OFC, and PCC are associated with self-referential processing, self-focus, and a bias towards negative emotional processing. Inability to deactivate PCC in cognitive activity interferes with cognitive control and mood regulation. (See Networks above)

With volume reduction in vmPFC and OFC, those with MDD, experience enhanced sensitivity to pain, and this reduction, is associated with Anxiety and ruminating thoughts.

Ruminative responses to negative life events involve the Posterior Cingulate Cortex.

Key Limbic Reflex Areas for Depression

Hippocampus and Subiculum. Reduced volume of the Hippocampus. SSRIs are thought to reverse this reduction.

HPA. Depression is often accompanied by Anxiety, loss of appetite, insomnia and reversed circadian rhythms.

sgACC. Loss of connection with the Amygdala.

Amygdala. Reduced regulation.

OFC, Striatum and NAc. Involved in reward circuits. Aversive mode associated with anhedonia and social withdrawal.

Locus Coeruleus. Reduced arousal and retarded activity.

Insula. Stress and emotional responses.

It has been suggested that in MDD, on assuming cognitive task behaviours, there is a malfunction in the switching between networks. The DMN is not getting switched off so there is a continuation of ruminating thought, which impacts on the ability to function in task related behaviours.

Post Trauma Stress

Now we have looked at how memories are formed, stored, retrieved and processed, we are able to explore post-traumatic stress, and the disorder PTSD, which involve problems in the processes involved in episodic or autobiographical memory.

The symptoms can be grouped into three categories:

- Intrusive thoughts.
- Avoidance behaviour and numbing.
- Hyperarousal.

Anyone may develop features of post trauma stress. They may become hypervigilant or have intrusive thoughts about the event. Following a traumatic event, not everyone will develop PTSD. In fact, only around 10% of those experiencing or witnessing life-threatening events, develop the disorder.

For most people, the reaction is transient. So why do some, and not others, develop PTSD? How someone responds to a stressor depends on:

- the nature of the trauma.
- personal experience.
- biological factors.
- genetic factors.

As an example, one finding shows that disrupted or delayed neural development influences the response to trauma. Children who have suffered abuse or had childhood trauma, are not only more susceptible to PTSD in later life, but also to a wide range of emotional disorders. It has been found that childhood trauma affects the normal development of the Hippocampus, thus rendering them more prone to mood disorders, Anxiety, and PTSD.

The difference between post trauma stress and PTSD concerns the range and intensity of reactions and the length of time that these continue to disrupt normal functioning.

Post-traumatic stress is only classified as a disorder if the presentation meets very stringent criteria. The most widely used criteria are those defined by the Diagnostic and Statistical Manual (DSM). We use these criteria to measure outcomes of treatment for PTSD.

Neurobiology of PTSD

In PTSD, there is altered function in all our players

Insula

- Smaller Left Insula.
- Increased activation, dysfunctional saliency role.
- Greater bilateral Insula responsivity to pain.
- increased Insula activation during the anticipation of negative versus positive.

Amygdala

- Increased activation and hyper-responsive.
- Less regulated (sgACC, Hippocampus).
- It also initiates the fear startle response, which is an exaggerated response to auditory and visual stimuli. This fear startle response is a major feature of PTSD. (This involves the PAG).

Hippocampus

- Reduced Hippocampus volume. It is unclear whether the smaller volume in PTSD is a predisposing factor or an effect of PTSD.
- Decreased function and activation.
- The Hippocampus is involved in the context of fear memory.

Locus Coeruleus

- Hyperactive in PTSD.
- Involved in encoding of fear memories. Norepinephrine from LC maintains LTP for context fear memory in the Hippocampus.
- Phasic phase involved in hypervigilance, a cardinal feature of PTSD and poor concentration.

Striatum & Nucleus Accumbens

- Less active.
- Loss of motivation in seeking positive rewards.
- Focus on avoiding negative rewards.
- Social detachment.

sgACC

- Smaller sgACC (the anterior Subgenual ACC is concerned with emotional regulation and the posterior with Infralimbic control over Amygdala.)
- Decreased activation.

HPA axis

- Some studies indicate reduced Cortisol and flattened daily variation in PTSD.
- Hypersensitive negative feedback loop, so reduced CRH and less ACTH. To compound this, there is a blunted ACTH sensitivity to CRH which all leads to reduced Cortisol production by the Adrenals.
- CRH plays a role in extinction of fear memory, hence the problems with extinction of fear memory.

BNST

- Altered balance of inhibiting and promoting influence, leading to hypervigilance and heightened cued anxiety.

Fibromyalgia

Fibromyalgia is a non-inflammatory syndrome where there is chronic widespread pain at multiple tender points, with no clear underlying organic disease.

It is accompanied by a wide range of problems including joint stiffness, mood disorders, low energy and fatigue, cognitive dysfunction, ('fibro fog'), and sleep disturbance. Irritable Bowel Syndrome (IBS) and migraine are also common in those suffering with Fibromyalgia.

Evidence suggests several processes are involved, in Fibromyalgia.

- Widespread Central Sensitisation.
- Increased activation of the Insula – sensory amplification.
- Reduced Dopamine release from the basal ganglia (Substantia Nigra).
- Reduced descending analgesia – decreased binding of mu receptors.
- Reduced activity in PAG – loss of inhibitory controls.
- Impaired inhibitory pathway with reduced Serotonin (Raphe underfunction), with abnormally high levels of Substance P.
- Reduced Norepinephrine – loss of inhibitory control at spinal cord and reduced enhancement of opiates.
- Reduced connections between ACC and Hippocampus, Amygdala and Thalamus.
- Thalamus under-functioning and sensitised.

- Under active HPA axis with a CRH deficiency from the Hypothalamus.
- Atrophy of the Adrenals due to chronic under-stimulation, aggravated by reduced ACTH levels.
- Sensitisation of Nucleus Accumbens.
- Immune system involvement.

Looking at this list, it is evident that Limbic Reflexology is ideally suited to Fibromyalgia. Indeed, much of the development of Limbic Reflexology involved working with those living with the condition.

The aim of treatments is to improve function. Generally, six to eight weekly treatments are required initially, followed by maintenance treatments monthly.

Myalgic Encephalomyelitis

Myalgic Encephalomyelitis (M.E.), is a complex autoimmune condition.

It involves a wide range of dysfunctional processes.

- Pain.
- Central Sensitisation.
- Fatigue.
- Hypocortisolaemia.
- HPA underactive. Pituitary feedback loop compromised.
- Adrenal insufficiency.
- Immune involvement.
- Often history of early trauma and mononucleosis.
- Reactivation of the Epstein Barr Virus (EBV).
- Oxidative stress.

For an interesting and informative overview of ME, read the Jason article on Kindling. Link to this on the student area on the website.

Irritable Bowel Syndrome

In IBS, changes in the gastrointestinal tract influence the brain through the Brain Gut Axis (BGA), and this alters the motility of the gut and activates the immune system.

Changes observed in IBS;

- Thinning of the Anterior Cingulate Cortex (ACC).
- Increased grey matter in the Hypothalamus.
- ACC, Insula, PFC, Striatum and Thalamus are all more activated than normal.
- Deficiencies in white matter in ACC and Insula.
- Deficiencies in descending pain pathways.
- Impaired Hippocampus.
- Immune function in the gut is hypersensitive, which leads to low level inflammation and more degranulated mast cells. All this activates BGA.
- Exaggerated response to pain.

There is also a link between fear and the sensitivity of the bowel. The link is the Amygdala, leading to significant activation of the Hypothalamus, ACC, PFC, and PAG. Fear and anxiety increase the action of the sympathetic nervous system which in turn increases the motility in the gut. Serotonin, synthesised in the gut wall, is the main neurotransmitter involved in peristalsis. Therefore, SSRI antidepressants, which increase the available Serotonin, can have the side effect of increased gut motility.

So, in IBS, we would work all the limbic reflex areas and lymphatic reflex areas.

Neuropathic Pain and Complex Regional Pain Syndrome

Most commonly involving a limb. Although the initial injury may be resolved, there has been damage to a nerve. Symptoms include Allodynia, Hyperalgesia, and restricted lifestyle functioning.

- There is atrophy of the Insula, and PFC.
- Contralateral activation of the Nucleus Accumbens, that is, the Nucleus Accumbens is activated on the opposite side of the injury.
- In CRPS, evidence suggests that the inhibitory pain pathways are compromised, resulting in reduced Serotonin and Norepinephrine.
- Dysfunctional Locus Coeruleus contributes to development of Allodynia, or over-sensitivity to, normally neutral stimulation.
- There is a specific area of the posterior Insula associated with Allodynia.
- In CRPS, the activated alpha1 receptors (pain increase), overwhelm alpha2 receptors (inhibitory), at the level of the spinal cord.
- There is reduced Hippocampal volume in neuropathic pain. This reduced volume may be associated with development of Depression, common in chronic pain.

Chronic Back Pain

In chronic back pain there is diverse atrophy of brain regions. PFC and OFC are especially involved. It is sensitised to continuous negative evaluations, enhanced by periodic pain signals.

The perceived level of pain is often disproportionate to the degree of injury.

Osteoarthritis

This is a degenerative joint condition, with damage to bone and cartilage.

There is widespread atrophy (reduction in volume) of brain regions.

Pain severity is proportionate with the extent of the damage but pain intensity is not, which suggests central sensitisation with lowered pain thresholds and hyperalgesia.

There is increased activation of the pain facilitatory pathway.

Rheumatoid Arthritis

Rheumatoid Arthritis is an autoimmune disease with systemic inflammation. As in Fibromyalgia, there is lowered Serotonin and Norepinephrine.

These deficiencies impair the descending pain inhibitory pathways.

The functions of both the PFC and the ACC are specifically impaired.

Glossary

Below is a brief glossary of some of the terms and concepts you may encounter on reading scientific articles.

Contralateral - opposite side.

Ipsilateral - same side.

Co-morbidity - suffering from one condition, at the same time as another. e.g. IBS is often a co morbid condition, in Fibromyalgia.

Atrophy - reduction in volume or wasting.

Attenuate - to reduce or lessen.

Mediate - involved in the process, or is the catalyst in, a process.

Rostral - towards the beak, or nose.

Ventral- towards the stomach, or below.

Dorsal - on the back, or top.

Caudal - towards the tail.

Appendix A

Medication commonly prescribed for chronic pain conditions.

Tramadol is a weak opioid with combined μ-receptor agonist and also a Serotonin and a Norepinephrine Reuptake Inhibitor, thus encouraging pain inhibition through the effects of Noradrenaline.

Duloxetine is licensed in some countries for Fibromyalgia. It is a SNRI, which means that it is a Serotonin <u>and</u> a Norepinephrine Reuptake Inhibitor, thus increasing the availability of both. It has a five-fold stronger effect on serotonin than on norepinephrine.

This is designed to compensate for impaired descending analgesic pathways. Duloxetine is licensed in the US, for the treatment of Fibromyalgia.

Tricyclics, such as Amitriptyline, are norepinephrine reuptake inhibitors but have more adverse side effects than SSRI's. It is sedative, so usually taken at night.

Gabapentin and Pregabalin, are medications originally used in the treatment of epilepsy. As the 'gaba' bit of their name suggests, they enhance the effects of GABA, which we know to have an inhibitory effect in the brain. They work in slightly different ways.

Pregabalin is much more potent (and much more expensive) Both medications however, can lead to significant weight gain.

Check Your Understanding.

What is the primary role of the limbic brain? (p1)

Name the three parts of the brainstem. (p4)

What are the three types of neuron? (p8)

What is the function of dendrites? (p9)

What cells form the myelin in the Central Nervous System? (p10)

What are nodes of Ranvier and what effect do they have on the speed of impulse transmission? (p10)

What effect does myelin have on a nerve impulse? (p10)

What is the function of receptors? (p15)

What is the main inhibitory neurotransmitter in the brain? (p19)

What are the different functions between the anterior and posterior Insula? (p23)

What area is involved in awareness of body states, and the intensity of pain? (p24)

What type of memories are stored in the Amygdala? (p28)

What is the main neurotransmitter synthesised in the Locus Coeruleus? (p35)

What nucleus in the Striatum influences motivation and goal seeking? (p45)

What is the role of the infralimbic cortex? (p49)

How many pairs of nuclei are in the Hypothalamus? (p53)

Name a neurohormone. (p55)

What is the name of the 'master clock' in the Hypothalamus? (p59)

What reflex area is especially relevant in chronic or sustained Anxiety? (p64)

Where would we find the Rostral Cingulate Zone? (p76)

What is stress? (p85)

What pituitary hormone's synthesis is stimulated by CRH from the Hypothalamus? (p87)

Name the two adrenal hormones whose production is stimulated by ACTH? (p87)

Name two effects of Cortisol (p89)

Why does chronic stress slow down healing? (p89)

How do negative feedback loops regulate the HPA axis? (p91)

Name two adverse effects of chronic Cortisol secretion. (p95)

Name two effects of synaptic plasticity. (p101)

What is long-term potentiation? (p102)

Name the four processes of memory formation. (p103)

When does a memory trace become labile and changeable? (p105)

What is the purpose of pain? (p111)

How does C fibres differ from A-delta fibres? (p114)

What is gateway inhibition? (p118)

Where is most of the brain's Serotonin produced? (p119)

At the level of the spinal cord, how does Serotonin influence pain signalling? (p119)

What brainstem nucleus is involved in both the facilitation of pain and its inhibition? (p120)

Where are endogenous endorphins mainly synthesised? (p123)

What nuclei are involved in attention to pain? (p125)

How do emotional states influence the perception of pain? (p126)

What is meant by central sensitisation? (p134)

What network assesses the significance of incoming information? (p139)

Limbic Reflexology Courses

Following the publication of this Textbook in 2016, there has been widespread interest in Limbic Reflexology from around the world, with enquiries about training opportunities. The online version of the course is in response to this interest.

For details about both the in-person courses and Limbic Reflexology Online, visit the Limbic Reflexology website.

https://limbicreflexology.com/

Index

ACC *76, 123, 125, 128, 130, 134, 137, 140, 153, 156, 159*

Addiction...*45, 64, 81*

ADHD *44, 71, 74, 77*

Adrenal Glands *89*

Allodynia... **132**

aMCC **75**, *137*

Amygdala.... **27**, *30, 49, 50, 63, 91, 100, 106, 110, 119, 126, 128, 132, 143, 147, 150, 156*

Anxiety............. *33, 37, 47, 58, 63, 64, 81, 85, 126,* **143**, *146, 147, 150, 152, 156*

BNST **63**, *65, 91, 152*

Brain Gut Axis *92*

Central Executive Network... **140**

Central Sensitisation *132,* **134**, *153, 155, 159*

Cerebellum.. **83**

Chronic Back Pain **158**

Chronic Pain *29, 40, 111, 112, 119, 124, 125, 127, 128, 131,* **132**, *133, 134, 135, 141, 146, 163*

Cingulate..**73**, *128, 139*

Classical Conditioning **99**

Corpus Callosum *49,* **78**, *146*

Cortisol... **89**

Default Mode Network **139**

Depression *19, 24, 32, 33, 34, 37, 45, 81, 86, 134, 141,* **145**, *146, 147, 157*

Descending Analgesia................................. *67, 69, 119,* **123**, *132, 153*

Embodied Cognition.. **98**

Emotions **97**

Fear Memory *67, 109, 130, 151, 152*

Fibromyalgia.. **153**

General Adaptation Syndrome **93**

Habenula *4,* **81**

Hippocampus *28,* **31**, *32, 33, 60, 64, 76, 79, 91, 94, 95, 104, 105, 106, 107, 110, 128, 134, 139, 143, 147, 151, 156*

HPA Axis... **87**

HPA feedback loop.. **91**

Hyperalgesia..**132**, *133, 157, 159*

Hypothalamus **53**, *63, 87, 93, 119, 123, 134, 141, 142, 154, 156*

Insula **23**, *125, 126, 128, 130, 134, 137, 139, 140, 147, 150, 153, 156, 157*

Irritable Bowel Syndrome **156**

LHA **57**, *141*

Locus Coeruleus ...**35**, *91, 101, 107, 120, 123, 125, 131, 137, 141, 147, 151, 157*

Mammillary Bodies **60**
Memory 31, 44, 49, 60, **99**
    consolidation 104
    encoding 104
    episodic **103**
    retrieval 105
    'Sins' of memory 105
    storage... 104
    types of memory.. 103
Mindfulness and Meditation.. 137
Myalgic Encephalomyelitis... **155**
Myelin Sheath **10**
Neurons.. **8**
Neuropathic Pain 37, **157**
Neurotransmitters **16**
Nociception **113**, 115, 117
Nucleus Accumbens **45**, 47, 71, 147
OCD 37, 44, 45, 49, 75, 105
OFC **47**, 75, 134, 147, 158
Operant Conditioning.. **100**
Osteoarthritis... **159**
PAG **67**, 68, 69, 106, 132, 141, 150, 153, 156
Pain.....................24, 25, 28, 29, 36, 40, **111**, 147, 150, 153, 155, 156, 163, 165
Pain Inhibition...19, 36, **118**, 163
Parkinson's Disease...17, 19, 37, 44, 71
PCC... **74**, 140, 147
Pineal 4, 54, 59, **82**, 142
Pituitary **51**, 54, 87, 123, 129, 155
Post Trauma Stress **149**
Preoptic... **56**, 61, 141
PVN **55**
Raphe..**69**, 81, 119, 133, 153
RCZ... **76**
Receptors **15**
Reuniens.. **79**
Rheumatoid Arthritis.. **159**
Saliency Network **139**
SCN..**59**, 82, 141, 142
sgACC... 49, 50, 63, 64, 147, 150, 151
Sleep **141**
Stress Response.. **87**
Striatum.......................... 40, **43**, 44, 71, 76, **129**, 134, 147, 151, 156
Subiculum **34**, 91, 129, 147
Substantia Nigra 44, **71**, 153
Synapse.. **11**

Synaptic Plasticity **101**
Thalamus *4, 23, **39**, 40, 60, 79, 117, 128, 134, 146, 153, 156*
TMN *56, **58**, 141*
VTA **71**, 81*
Wind up and Summation *133*

172